Learning now to Land

Sketches from a year in community health

Jim Clayton

Dedicated with love and respect
to the staff of the NHS.

Contents

The following sketches are taken from my experiences as a nursing assistant within a community health team. Some details have been changed to protect patient confidentiality.

Who we are

'Do you know who we are? Has anyone told you what we do?'

I say it a lot. I'm like an actor in a long-running play, trying to find novelty in lines I've said so many times they've picked up a disreputable shine.

'We're an NHS community health team. Nurses, physios, occupational therapists... you name it! A small bank of emergency carers. Even a pharmacist!'

I like putting that in. Makes us sound like a friendly high street. All the usual shops.

'We work on a pretty tight schedule – just three days – and our job is to support patients being discharged from hospital, or help stop them being admitted in the first place. If longer term stuff is needed, we refer on to the District Nurses or the specialist teams like the Respiratory or Heart Failure people. We're basically another emergency service...'

A great many of the patients we see are struggling. But although the specifics of each situation change, the basics stay the same: they can't cope, and they need help to get back to coping. There is a phrase you see a lot in the paperwork: *Back to baseline* – a simple expression that neatly caps a world of negotiation, delicate interventions, difficult decisions, compromise.

Back to Baseline.

'Any questions?'

1: Dogs

'Are you okay with dogs?'

It's an article of faith to say yes, because Leila's brindle Staffie Frankie is hurling himself against the baby gate so violently you'd think he hadn't eaten in a week and a leg of mutton just walked in the door.

Before I can answer either way, Leila unlatches the gate and Frankie bursts out. I stand my ground and ignore him – and, thank god, it works. In fact, it's extraordinary how quickly he changes mode: from Hound of Hell to Snuffling Chump.

I scraggle him behind the ears, and he seems to like that. Then suddenly he's reminded of something and hurries off into the sitting room.

'Oh no,' says Leila. 'Wait for it.'

There's a plaintive squeak or two, then Frankie comes trotting back into the hallway to sit at my feet with a blue ball clamped in his jaws.

'Oh for God's sake,' says Leila. 'Him and that ball. I wish I'd never got it.'

Frankie bites down on it twice in quick succession, to emphasise.

'It was funny the other night, though,' says Leila. 'He fell asleep with it in his mouth. Then he started dreaming, doing that spooky eye-rolling thing they do, twitching and jerking, and then the ball squeaked, and woke him up, and scared the bejeesus out of him. He fell off the sofa and the ball squeaked some more and he dropped it and ran behind the curtains. I thought that might've cured him. But no, he was straight back on it. Poor ol' Frankie. He's like me – an addictive personality.'

There is a middle-aged man and woman, standing side-by-side at the living room window of the bungalow next door, staring at me as I walk down the path. I wave – as best I can with all the bags I'm carrying –

3

but they don't wave back. It wouldn't surprise me if they were actually cut-outs, set there by an estate agent. But if that's true, why not give them wavy arms and flashing eyes, activated by a sensor when you got close enough? As it is, their bungalow looks about as homey and real as a house made of Lego. Even the juniper in the planter wears a tag.

Mind you, the bungalow I'm visiting has more than enough reality for both. A low, brick wall separates the two of them as severely as the line between a 'Before' and 'After' feature. It's a wretched, tumbledown affair, with an overgrown garden, rotten woodwork, missing tiles, and a car parked round the back, one of those boaty old Citroens, crusted in mould, the bonnet disappearing into the tarmac like a junk submarine in the world's slowest dive.

I glance over my shoulder. The cut-outs have been repositioned to get a better look.

I put my stuff down, reach out, and knock.

The instantaneous and outraged barking of a dog.

Scuffling, swearing, crashing – the sounds of a desperate struggle in the hallway. I guess the dog is being put in a cage; if it is, it only makes the barking worse, like trying to stuff a panther in a cereal box.

After a composing kind of moment, the door opens. George stands there, breathing hard, pushing his hair back from his face, smiling, whilst a small terrier tries to cut through the bars with acetylene fury.

'Don't mind Trampus,' says George. 'He's very protective.'

'I'd never have guessed he was a terrier!'

'Well. He's crossed with something bigger.'

'A wolf?'

'Possibly. In his head.'

'I don't mind if you let him out. I'm alright with dogs.'

George's smile tightens.

'Oh, no,' he says. 'Oh, no, no, no. I couldn't possibly.'

As if to illustrate, Trampus redoubles his efforts, the cage rocking from side to side.

'Well. Alright then,' I say.

'Thank you for coming,' says George, backing up.

4

George is as friendly, nub-faced, vast and shiningly white as a beluga whale, his trousers suspended by hoops, the lenses of his glasses thumbed with grease. He leads me back through the house, which is just as awful as the outside promised, comprehensively silted up with trash in the hoarder-style, unwashed plates stacked in plastic buckets, strata of food trodden into the floor. Even though it's early in the year, a couple of plump black flies are on the move. One buzzes past me in a straight line from Crap A to Crap B, somnolent and satisfied as a bank manager on the daily commute.

'Mother? There's a gentleman to see you. From the hospital.'

'Hello Gladys. My name's Jim. How are you today?'

Gladys is as thin as George is fat. A frail and spidery old woman in a housecoat and flowery bandana, she's not sitting in her chair so much as nesting in it, kyphotically hunched over a plate of digestives, scooping up the pieces and pressing them into her whiskery mouth.

'Trampus has gone quiet,' I say, looking for somewhere to put my bags, not finding anywhere.

'Eerily quiet,' says George.

'What's he doing? Tunnelling?'

'Oh no!' says George. 'Don't say that.'

Billy is thin and white like forced celery, wisps of white hair streaming back from his chiselled forehead against all natural gravitational laws, his etiolated white hands clasping the armrests of the chair like roots he put out to suck the nutrients from the stuffing. He barely acknowledges me as I let myself in. Whether that's because of a general remoteness, or because he's drunk most of the various spirit bottles placed artfully around his feet, it's hard to tell.

'How come you didn't answer your phone, Billy?'

He turns his sad blue eyes up to me.

'Oh. Was that you ringing? I looked for my phone but I couldn't find it.'

'Shall I give it another ring and see where it is?'

He shrugs.

I go to recents in my phone, and call.

After a moment, a loud buzzing starts up on the cluttered table immediately in front of us. His phone is under a red reminder.

'Found it!'

'Great' he says, in a whispery voice leached flat by long hours of nothing in particular. 'Gis it here, then.'

It's hard to know what to do about Billy. The best you can say is that he has a workmanlike approach to drinking himself to death. There's no joy in it; no wild ride. For some reason he's simply hitched himself to a slow and monotonous decline, slumped in an armchair that's sinking beneath a quicksand of liquor bottles. When the glass level reaches the bridge of his nose, I don't imagine he'll struggle. He'll merely turn those eyes in the direction of whoever's there to notice, and gently slide out of sight with a clink.

I unzip my bag and loop the stethoscope round my neck. When I straighten, I notice the four dog photos taped to the wall on his right. The photos have been printed A4 size with the colour running low, so everything's a little fuzzy. You can see it's the same dog, though, a lugubrious hound sitting in the same position in the kitchen, wearing four different hats: a fisherman's floppy cap; a Norwegian-style knitted hat with flaps; a panama, and then something from a fancy dress shop – a plastic policeman's helmet fastened under its chin with elastic.

'Love the pictures!' I tell him. 'Whose dog is that?'

'Karen, my carer,' Billy whispers, sadly. 'She knows I like dogs. And hats.'

❧

Millie's poodle Rosie bounds off the sofa when I come in. She lies with her paws either side of a well-chewed rubber Bugs Bunny, glancing down at it, then up to me, then down to the rabbit again, daring me to take it. I can't decide who has the maddest expression: the rabbit or the dog.

6

'I think… she thought… you were Janet,' says Millie. 'Janet… the dog walker.'

Millie furniture-walks to a seat at the dining room table. COPD has blasted her body, robbing her of any spare flesh. It's left her tentative and frail, spindle-thin as a giant crane fly, fumbling for purchase, somewhere to land and catch her breath and think about the day.

'I don't want much,' she wheezes. 'I've got… the medication I need… plus a little something… for anxiety. What I really need… is someone… to come in now and again… to help me… with a bath. That's all. Do my back… y'know?… the awkward bits.'

The doorbell rings and a breezy woman swathed in waterproofs stamps into the kitchen. I'm guessing it's Janet.

'Hiya Millie!' she says. 'Phew! It's bad out there. Oh! You've got company!'

I introduce myself, get up to shake her hand which is ice cold.

'You need gloves,' I say.

'I need a lot of things,' she says, pulling out a hankie and blowing her nose so loudly I take an involuntary step backwards. 'I need to win the lottery,' she says.

Meanwhile, Rosie has ditched the rabbit and dashed through to greet her. Janet kneels on the kitchen floor with her arms wide. Rosie puts her paws on the woman's knees so she can reach up and lick her face.

'You silly girl!' she says. 'I've had a wash today. I don't need another one. Do I? Hey?'

'Will… she be… alright?' says Millie. 'It looks… pretty bad out there.'

'Of course!' says the woman, grasping the kitchen counter, struggling to get up again. 'Oof!'

She looks at me.

'Got any spare knees in your bag?'

'I'll have a look.'

'Good boy.'

She reaches into her pocket for a treat, and for a moment I think she's going to throw it to me. But Rosie sits excitedly at her feet, and Janet hands it down to her instead.

'She'll be fine,' the woman says. 'It's so windy out, I'm thinking of tying some string round her legs and flying her like a kite.'

Millie gives her a panicked look.

'Seriously, though, we'll just go for a short one round the park,' says Janet, giving me such an exaggerated, lop-sided wink, I'm guessing her face is still numb from the cold.

❧

Rita is sitting in a high-backed chair watching a veterinary programme on television. A cow is so bloated the vet is driving a cannula fat as a marlinspike into its abdomen; the farmer and his wife put their hands over their noses. 'She'll be a lot more comfortable now,' the vet says. They nod, keeping their hands in place.

The television is on so loud Rita hasn't heard us come in, so as gently as I can, I say Good Morning and move into her line of sight.

She screams.

I've met Rita before, and I'd told Andreas, the physiotherapist who's come with me, what to expect. It's a particularly terrifying scream, though, and he visibly reddens.

'It's okay! It's okay!' he says. 'We're from the hospital. We've just come to see how you are and what you might need.'

She screams again – exactly the kind of sound effect you'd want in a horror film if an elderly person was being murdered. Such an open-throated, desperate noise, made worse by the slack cavity of her mouth and the two, blockish teeth, offset top and bottom.

The odd thing is, she's not screaming because we've scared her coming into the flat. She's screaming because she wants us to do something. And sure enough, when I ask what it is, she points to the kitchen trolley.

'The remote? You want me to pass you the remote?'

She screams again.

8

'There you are, Rita! And please try very hard not to scream like that if you can, because it makes it difficult to understand what you're after.'

'Thank you,' she says, in a normal voice, and stuffs the remote into the cushion beside her on the chair.

Andreas looks shaken, but I think he's reassured I'm not freaking out. He adopts a calm, super-moderate tone.

'Now then, Rita,' he says, squatting down and resting a hand on hers. 'I'm the physiotherapist, and you've met Jim before, the nursing assistant. Is it okay if we ask you a few questions to find out how we can help you after your stay in hospital? Would that be alright?'

She fishes out the remote control with her free hand and raps him on the knuckles with it – I guess because he's in the way of her vet programme.

'Oh! Sorry!' he says, rubbing his hand and standing up again. 'But Rita – would you mind if we turned the television down a little bit? So we wouldn't have to shout?'

She screams again, and he almost falls over.

'Now, now!' I say. 'Come on, Rita! Remember what we said about the screaming? Try to tell us as calmly as you can what it is you want.'

'Soup!' she says. 'I want soup!'

'Okay. That's okay. I'll make you some soup,' says Andreas, 'but first let's get the assessment out of the way, shall we?'

She turns off the TV and grumpily stuffs the remote into the chair cushion again.

Andreas has just turned his back to open his folders when she screams again, so loudly he almost dumps the lot on the floor.

'What is it now?' he says.

'Clean these!' she shouts, handing him two filthy magnifying lenses. 'Clean them!'

'Okay. I'll rinse them under the tap for you, but then I really must get on with my paperwork. Okay?'

He takes the glasses, shakes his head at me, then goes into the kitchen.

9

'Whilst Andreas is doing that, d'you mind if I take your blood pressure and so on?'

She grunts, staring at the television.

A rabbit is being sedated prior to an operation. The vet says he'll take this opportunity to clip its nails, too.

I approach with my kit, gently wrapping a blood pressure cuff round her arm, and then putting the steth in my ear. Just behind her I notice a yellowing, photocopied picture taped to the wall – a Welsh terrier, sitting with its paws on a table. The dog is wearing pince-nez specs, a red spotted neckerchief and a knitted waistcoat. 'He's lovely,' I say, nodding at the picture. 'What's his name?'

Rita screams.

It's completely heart-stopping, like I've put the stethoscope into the mouth of a roaring lion. I snatch it clear and take a step back.

'What?' I say, shakily.

'A girl!' she says, in her normal voice. 'She was a girl'.

Then she picks up the remote control, points it at the TV, and turns it up, full volume.

Angus, the focus of all this Scottie dog memorabilia, is lying on his tummy on a Scottie dog patterned rug. I'm relieved that he IS a Scottie dog, otherwise everything surrounding him – the Scottie dog toy in the white plastic alcove hung with fairy lights; the hundreds of Scottie dog pictures hanging on the walls, some as hyper-colourised 3D versions, where the eyes open and the tongue lolls out as you pass; the Scottie dog tea-towels neatly draped on a rail; the Scottie dog biscuit tin, the Scottie dog cushions, the Scottie dog puzzle half-completed on the table, with (ominously) only the eyes to complete – well, if you walked into a flat like this and found a Doberman, you'd probably lose your mind.

'Don't go near him,' says Jean. 'He bites.'

'He's so sweet,' I say.

'Only when he's sleeping,' says Melanie, Jean's daughter. 'He bites me, too.'

'Oh.'

'I wonder what he dreams about?' says Jean, yawning.

'Biting,' says Melanie.

I go to put my things down. Angus looks up. He's so old, his fur has a rubbed, slightly greasy look.

'Fifteen,' says Jean, anticipating my question.

'Wow! Fifteen! Well!' I say – then after a pause, where I can't actually bring myself to say that he looks good for fifteen, I manage instead: 'We've got a dog.'

'Oh yeah? What sort?'

'A lurcher.'

'How old?'

'I think she's about ten.'

'Ah!' says Jean. 'Long-legged dogs. They don't live long.'

'No. I've heard that.'

Angus may have lifted his head, but that's as much as he's prepared to do.

'Angus! GET over here!' says Melanie.

'Oh – he's alright' I say. Too late. Melanie has already pushed herself clear of the sofa. She reaches down to scoop him up, and immediately his eyes spring open, revealing two black buttons of insanity. He bares his teeth, as thin and brown and horribly curved as the teeth on a deep-sea angler fish, and he begins paddling furiously with his paws to turn and tear a lump out of her arm. It's a horrifying spectacle, like watching someone pick up a scatter cushion and finding it transformed into a demon.

'Oh no you don't, you little bastard' says Melanie, expertly wrestling Angus into a non-biteable position, and then sinking back onto the sofa with him, where she smothers the dog into submission. Eventually he taps out with a paw, Melanie cautiously relaxes her hold and Angus sits there huffing and gasping and catching his breath, all the while watching me with an expression of the purest hatred.

'Good boy,' says Jean.

Lucky's a hard man.

You can tell immediately – not so much from the ruin of his body, his arms and shoulders the texture of old stilton, veined and nicked and scabbed from years of drug abuse; not from his ill-fitting false teeth, his gold chains or his blurry tattoos – hula hula girl, flaming skull, Ace of Spades; nor from the casually terrible things he says, stories of violence, vendettas, feuds, armed robberies and the like. And it's not something you'd simply extrapolate from the block-cap note in the front of his folder: DOUBLE-UP VISITS IN THE PRESENCE OF SUPPORT WORKERS ONLY. No. Without any of these things you'd still be able to tell. He carries it deep in his eyes – an unsettling, milky blue, as if the poison of all that hostility rose up over the years and leached out the purer colour. I can imagine him turning those eyes on the face of enemy, warden or wall with the same languorously hostile expression. For now, though, he seems to have accepted my role in this particular scenario, and offers out his paw for the SATS probe with the weighty insouciance of a tiger, claws retracted.

'The doctor? Nah mate! They don't send doctors out to me no more. The last one, he said Your old man's very ill. Oh yes? I said. What the fack's wrong with the ol' cant now? I'm afraid he's got cancer he said. He's not got long to live. Is that right? I said. So I knocked him out...'

'The hardest thing about doing time's the first week. Once you done that it's easy. Piece of piss. You get in the routine, know what I mean? I've done plenty. Most of my life I've been one place or the other. You name it, I'll tell you the craic. I could write a book. Anyway, where I come from, half of us end up inside. Walking round the block was like walking round the old manor...'

'I think the worst thing they ever did was cut down on the heroin.

They jes' went an' made a whole lot of work for themselves. No-one's going to make any trouble smacked out of their heads, are they? Now they got all this other gear going in, fake stuff that winds you up and makes you punchy. You don't want that when you're all banged up, d'you? Stands to reason. But they don't think like that, do they?'

'I been in trouble since I was a kid. I got sent to borstal for stabbing up me eldest brother. I was ready to go and stab him up good n'proper when I got out, 'cept I was on a bank job and got sent down for a stretch before I got the chance. I haven't forgotten him though. Once these legs are better I'll be payin' the cant a little visit...'

Back in the support workers' office for the debrief, a mad-looking labradoodle is wandering round with a green and yellow plastic turtle. He goes from person to person, squeaking the toy a couple of times, dropping it at our feet, and then backing away with his mouth open and his tail wagging, looking up at our faces and then back down at the toy, as if he can't believe we're not as mad for it as he is.

'Buddy! Don't be such a pain!' says one of the support workers. She throws the toy for him anyway, and he races after it. After a while he brings it over to me, watching me with an insane expression as I pick it up and turn it over and over in my hands.

I have an image of Buddy behind bars, lights out, squeaking the turtle mournfully, like a harmonica.

I'm glad he's here, though. Buddy's like me. I don't think he'd cope all that well in prison, turtle or otherwise.

'There you go, Buddy!' I say, lobbing his toy back over the other side of the office.

He crashes after it.

∽

Each patient record has a reminder area on the home page. It's supposed to draw your attention to essential details or dangers, such as the need for double-up visits, the contact numbers of the relatives you must liaise with first, the keysafe code, any environmental dangers you should be aware of. So the first thing I write is:

Two small dogs – friendly, but bark when you knock

It's only when I read it back I see the problem with the sentence. So I delete and write instead:

Two small dogs. Loud to begin with, but soon settle down.

Mrs Albright is ninety-seven. She lives alone in a ramshackle bungalow, top of a narrow lane of cottages and heavily-buttressed flint walls leaning out at extraordinary angles, an ancient church under scaffolding, and a strange, round building with worn stones and arrow slits standing alone in a paddock, that looks like maybe it's the last thing standing of a castle, currently serving time as a chicken house.

Like most of everything else down the lane, Mrs Albright is old and falling down. But although physically she's reaching the end of her ability to cope, intellectually she's as formidable as ever.

'Apart from the carers coming in twice a day, and your family popping in when they can, do you manage to see anyone else?'

'Anyone else? Do you mean socially?'

'Well – yes, I suppose I do.'

'I run an ancient history group once a week, if that counts. Does that count?'

'I think that counts.'

'Excellent. Then – yes. Every Wednesday I have a dozen or so people round and we discuss a broad range of topics. Last Wednesday Sally did the Assyrians. This Wednesday it's Margaret on Alexander the Great.'

Whilst we're talking, Mrs Albright's dogs – two bug-eyed pugs – have plopped themselves down to sleep around her feet.

'Yes – I'm afraid they do that a lot,' she says, peering down. 'They like to be near me in case I drop anything overboard, a bit of crumpet or what have you, which I'm afraid to say does happen from time to time. The problem is I forget the damned things are there and when I get up to spend a penny, I go flying. It's a miracle I've lasted this long without breaking anything. Not so much as a cup.'

Mrs Albright's son Richard is sitting with us at the table. He's already mentioned that the family are looking at residential care, something Mrs Albright seems happy to think about.

'I'll miss the old place,' she says, planting both hands firmly on the table and looking around. 'But – you know, one thing that became very apparent to me very early on in my career, is that nothing lasts forever.'

∾⟨⟩

There's an extemporary, Mad Max feel to the front of the house, holes in the concrete forecourt filled in with rubble and crap, a derelict caravan green with mould dumped arse-first, blocking the sitting room windows, missing tiles in the path bridged with scraps of plasterboard, chipboard, whatever. It's like the occupants started scavenging a skip, then gave up, and went back inside.

I knock on the door.

Immediate, furious barking, shouting.

Eventually, from behind the glass: 'You alright with dogs, yeah?'

'Yep. Fine. It's okay.'

The door opens and someone throws an old, brindle-coloured footstool at me – that's what it feels like, at least – a footstool magically animated, with a tail and teeth and murderous intent.

'That's enough, Nipper! Let him alone now!'

Nipper wobbles up and down on his carved wooden legs, flapping his lid.

'Jes' ignore 'im,' says Thomas, waving me inside. 'He'll wear himself down eventually.'

Thomas takes his seat on a ruined sofa, in front of a TV showing Formula One. I put my bag down, and Nipper is all over it. If I'm not careful, he'll be running off down the road with my stethoscope trailing behind him, a cartoon dog with a string of sausages.

'I can put him outside if you like.'

'Nah. He's alright. It's nice to have an assistant.'

'Right'ya then.'

Thomas turns out to be an easy patient, if by easy you mean someone who doesn't want any help, and just wants to sit in all day, drinking and smoking.

'What's the use, fella? I appreciate you coming round n'all, but honestly – there are worse people out there. I don' wanna waste yer time.'

I ask him if he'd like me to make referrals to various people, for equipment and physiotherapy and so on, especially given his recent hospital admission and diagnosis. It all seems a bit pointless, though.

'Fair enough,' he says. 'It might be worth a punt.'

He stares down at his hands, listlessly massaging the palm of his right with the thumb of his left.

Nipper – who had retreated exhausted to his basket, suddenly leaps up and starts barking again, trampling straight over me in his eagerness to get to the front door. A second later the door opens, and a guy so huge steps in that the whole house seems to tilt in his direction.

'I'm Shaun, Thomas' son,' rumbles the guy, leaning down to shake my hand, making a real effort not to pick me up and shake the whole person by mistake. 'Everything alright with the ol' fella?'

'Yep. All good, considering. There are some things we could do to help – if he'll let us.'

'Hear that, da? Don't keep saying no to everything, would ya now?'

Thomas sneers and bats a hand in the air.

'Yah!' he says.

Shaun hesitates in the doorway, like he feels he should do more but can't think what. It's astonishing to think that Thomas is his father – not just the difference in size, but in vitality and sheer physical presence. I picture one of Thomas' sperm, scrub-chinned, spitty roll-up in the corner of its mouth, Stan Laurel twist of hair, idly corkscrewing its tail through the vulval gloom, by sheer blind accident driving its head before the thousands of others through the softly yielding wall of a certain egg.

'If you want me, I'll be in the van,' says Shaun.

I can't believe he means the ruin out front, but it's true. I see the shadow of it rock alarmingly as he goes inside. How it bears his weight I have no idea. Maybe when they go on holiday, he forces his legs through the floor, his arms through the window, and runs them all there.

'Do you like the ol' Formula One then?' says Thomas, nodding at the screen whilst he fishes his tobacco tin out from behind a cushion.

'I don't really follow it,' I tell him. 'I'd love to have a go, though.'

'What – driving one of dem things?' He grimaces, then attends to the business of rolling himself a fag, holding a paper between a thumb and two fingers, and then shakily losing half the tin of tobacco trying to fill it. 'Nah!' he says, giving up, rolling the fag ineffectually, running his tongue along the gummy strip. 'You gotta have nerves of steel for dem things.'

The moment I press the front bell, a furious howling and barking starts up deep within the house; a half second later, a malevolently dark shape starts leaping up and down the other side of the door, battering itself against the frosted butterfly glass, crazy as a baby wolf on a trampoline, doing everything it can to get to me bar setting up an oxy-acetylene cylinder and cutting a hole through the panel. A minute or so passes but the dog doesn't tire. It even seems to be trying out some fancy moves – a half-tuck, a forward roll. Eventually, a light goes on, and a shadow coalesces, three door panes into one.

'Shashi! Shashi! For goodness sake – shush now!' A chain rattles back, a lock turns, the door opens. Despite myself, I can't help drawing back, expecting the dog to launch itself at my throat; instead, it trots out quite happily to sniff my shoes, as if it was only contracted to bark so long as the door stayed shut.

'Lovely to see you!' says June. 'Sorry about Shashi. She sounds terrible but she's perfectly harmless.'

'Her bark's worse than her bite.'

'Well her bite's pretty bad, to be honest, but since she had her teeth out, she's calmed down in that respect.'

June leads me through to her living room. It's a tidy space, dominated right and left by two enormous Georgian-style doll's houses. Each house has a little patch of garden in front, surrounded by a white picket fence. In the garden of one, two elderly dolls lounge in deck chairs, reading the paper; in the other, a doll mows the lawn with a dog exactly like Shashi following behind.

'Have a seat,' says June. She gets into position to sit down herself, unaware that Shashi has already jumped up onto the armchair and – apparently – fallen asleep.

'Watch out!' I say.

'What? Oh – d'you mean the dog? She'll move.'

I can hardly watch.

June drops down into the chair immediately above the dog, which only moves at the very last second, reaching out with a paw to whip its tail out of the way as June lands with a weighty sigh.

'There!' she says. Then looks around.

'I don't know where the other is. They're thick as thieves, normally. Brother and sister. Peas in a pod.'

I'd spoken to June's son before coming here today. He'd talked to me about June's increasing problems with dementia, her loss of short-term memory, her habit of leaving the cooker on, door open, bath running. The whole thing is moving towards residential care, but for now the family were looking at increasing the number of carers during the day.

'It's been a difficult few days,' he'd said. 'Yesterday we had to have one of the dogs put down. The vet came out and it was pretty awful, but I'm not sure Mum remembers too much about it.'

I look over at Shashi. She's left June's armchair to curl up on one of two plush, tasselled red cushions on the opposite sofa. As if she can read my mind, she raises her head and stares at me.

'Don't!' she seems to say.

Avondale.

Sounds beautiful. Magical. I bet the architect was a fan of Lord of the Rings. You expect to see an ancient castle draped in moss and mist, with strange, long-legged birds circling and crying overhead, a plangent waterfall and so on, elfcetera, elfcetera. Instead what you get is an anonymous, prefab block just off the high street, tucked away behind a phony Italian restaurant. It's only been up a year or so but already it has a tired, beaten-down kind of look, strips of tape over the intercom where the buttons have fallen off. If the same architect had worked on Helm's Deep, I don't think Saruman would've needed much more than a couple of orcs and a wheelbarrow to tear the place down.

The one magical thing about Avondale, though, is its uncanny ability to screw up the SatNav. The app doesn't recognise the postcode at all, and ends up recommending you 'make a u-turn' and then 'make another
u-turn' so that if you were truly dependent on it, you'd end up simply driving in a circle at the bottom of the high street until you ran out of fuel or the police threw stingers down.

Cherry lives on the first floor with her little Jack Russell, Dave. Cherry has a long list of health problems, from mental health and self-harm to morbid obesity, diabetes, breathing problems and recurrent infections, and she's been referred to us many times in the past. She's got a reputation for being difficult, but I think because I make a fuss of Dave whenever I go there, she takes it easy on me.

'Cherry was pretty sick this time,' says Michela, the co-ordinator. 'She went in with an exacerbation of COPD, but then self-discharged against advice. She was so bad they gave her home oxygen. So can you pop-in, see how she's doing? Get her to sign a non-concordance form if necessary.'

Cherry is propped up in bed watching CSI. The first thing I notice – after Dave has finished leaping madly around my legs – is that Cherry's wearing a nasal cannula connected by a long, plastic tube that snakes across the bed to an oxygen cylinder by the window. The second thing I notice is the fag in her mouth.

'Erm … Cherry? You really can't be smoking when you're using oxygen.'

'What? Wha'dy'a mean?'

'You'll blow yourself up. And everyone else. You'll send Dave into orbit. Honestly, mate – you've got to put the fag out.'

She shrugs, pinches the end out, and rests it carefully on the ashtray by the bed.

'Thank you,' I say. 'I'm sorry to be so blunt about it, but you absolutely cannot smoke with oxygen around. This whole place'll go up.'

'I only have one now and again. It's not a problem.'

The heaped ashtray and the smoky fug in the room tell a different story. I know I'll have to report this to her GP and the Community Respiratory Team as soon as I'm back in the car, but for now I move on.

Dave is on the bed now. He rolls onto his back so I can rub his tummy, his tongue lolling out with the ecstasy of it all.

'So how've you been?' I say to Cherry. 'Sorry to hear about your recent hospital trip.'

'Yeah – well. What can you do? They said I had to go. I didn't want to. I mean – what are they going to do about anything?'

'I don't know, Cherry. But to be fair, they do seem to have done quite a bit. Put you on IV antibiotics, sent you for chest x-rays, got you back on your feet.'

'Yeah, but they didn't, did they? Look at me!'

'It says in your notes you self-discharged against advice. Is that right?'

She shrugs.

'They made it impossible. It was noisy. I couldn't sleep. They wake you up every five minutes to fiddle about. The nurses were rude. The food was unbelievable. I mean – you've got to be really sick to want to go to that place.'

'That's true. And from the sounds of it – I think you were pretty sick. And still are.'

I unclip the SATS probe from her finger.

'Your oxygen levels are terrible, Cherry – even for you. And that's five minutes after you came off the oxygen.'

'Yeah – and I'd still be on it if you hadn't said.'

'It's a choice, though, isn't it. No oxygen and low SATS, or oxygen and burst into flames. Isn't it, Dave? Isn't it…?'

Something suddenly occurs to him, because he flips himself upright again, hurls himself off the bed, and skitters off across the laminate flooring into the kitchen.

'Oh my God! Wait for it,' says Cherry.

There's a single, loud squeak from the kitchenette, and then Dave hurries back with a red, rubber bone in his mouth. It's so big he can't make it up on the bed again without a boost from me. As soon as he's there, though, he chows up and down on it, making it squeak as regularly as a monitor in a hospital for clowns.

I look down at Dave. 'God – it's noisier than the ward,' says Cherry. 'And before you say anything, I don't care, I'm not going back.'

'What do you think?' I ask him. 'What do you think mummy should do?'

He stares up at me, panting excitedly, flicking his eyes without moving his head… down to the bone… up to me … down to the bone… up to me.

'Dave says it's tricky.'

Lolly and Richard slot around each other like two old spoons. Or two pieces of an antique jigsaw (maybe 'Seaside View' or 'A Day at the Races'). Everything they do is coordinated. The way they move, for example. Even though it's a big house they seem to continually be in each other's way. When Lolly starts up the stairs, Richard wants to come down. When Lolly heads for the sitting room, Richard comes out. When Lolly goes into the kitchen to fetch something, Richard goes with her, so that when she turns round, she has to put her hands on his shoulders and manoeuvre past him in something that – from a safe distance – looks suspiciously like a dance. Their conversation is slotted, too. Their sentences run into each other. They finish what the other was saying. They snipe, but in such a practised and good-natured way, they're like two elderly vaudevillians whose routine is domestic war and loving irritation. They've been touring this show for so long now and they know their parts back to front. It's a job to see where one performer ends and the other begins.

They've got a dog, too. Willard – a Golden Retriever.

To begin with, I think it's Willard who answers the door when I ring. It's the way he paws it to one side, with such an open and happy expression I half-expect him to say Good Morning and How may I help? Instead, the door opens even wider and I see Lolly standing there.

'You're the nurse are you?' she says. 'Good. Maybe you can take him away. He's driving me mad.'

'Who is it Lolly? Who's there?'

'It's the nurse. Come to give you a brain transplant.'

'A brain transplant? Excellent. Ask him if he'll give you a heart at the same time.'

'Where do you want him?' says Lolly, sighing and looking back at me. 'I could give you a couple of suggestions.'

In the meantime, Richard has come halfway down the stairs.

'I'm easy,' I say. 'Wherever he's most comfortable.'

'He wants you in the bedroom,' says Lolly, putting a hand on the balustrade, as if she's going to stop him coming any further by main force.

'I'm glad somebody does.'

'Oh dear God,' says Lolly. She sighs. 'He's been a bit – you know – since the op.'

It's one of the reasons I've been asked to visit, to check the wound and make sure he hasn't got an infection. The GP has already given him some antibiotics, delivered remotely, as they often are these days. I wouldn't be surprised if next year they started using drones. Although – to be fair – looking at myself reflected in the hallway mirror – it looks like they already are.

Lolly starts up the stairs. There's a battle royale, Richard wanting to come down, Lolly telling him to reverse. I say I don't mind where. Richard says he wants the sitting room. Okay I say. No says Lolly. Reverse. Lie on the bed. Willard is right behind me, smiling broadly. The four of us continue up the stairs in one well-coordinated bundle.

'He's been hallucinating,' says Lolly, as Richard lies back on the bed.

'I have not,' he says.

'Yes you have, darling.'

'When?'

'This morning.'

'Why? What happened?'

'There!' says Lolly, nodding at me. 'Even his memory's going.'

'No, no!' says Richard, quite happily, adjusting the pillows behind his head and then folding his hands on his tummy. 'I'm simply disputing your version of events.'

'You said there was a big orange fish behind the telly.'

'Not was, darling. Is. There IS a big orange fish behind the telly.'

'You see,' says Lolly. 'D'you think it's serious?'

'Have a look for yourself!' says Richard.

'Oh for goodness sake.'

I go over to the telly.

'I hate to say this, Lolly – but there is actually a big orange fish down there.'

'Not you too... oh!'

We're both looking down at the gap behind the telly. There's a cuddly toy lying on the cables – a Finding Nemo clown fish.

'Well who put that there?' says Lolly.

Willard looks up at me with a broadly innocent look on his face. I'm immediately suspicious.

'Search me,' says Richard. 'Look – are we going to do this thing or not? Because quite frankly, I'm hungry and I want my kippers.'

'That's a good sign,' I say, turning back to the bed.

'Is it?' sighs Lolly. 'Is it?'

'All our dogs have started with a W,' says Lolly, as I tidy up my things. 'First there was Winston. Then it was Willow.'

'No, darling. No. It was Wilma after Winston. Then it was Willow.'

'You're quite right. Winston. Wilma. Willow. Willard.'

'I like that!' I say. 'How did it all start?'

'It was Lolly's idea,' says Richard.

'They've all been rescues,' says Lolly. 'We didn't like their names so we had to change them. Winston was easy, because his original name was Branston.'

'Like the pickle,' says Richard.

'Like the pickle,' says Lolly. 'We didn't like the idea of calling out Branston and immediately thinking of pickle. Neither of us likes pickle. So we wanted a name that sounded like Branston, so the dog wouldn't get confused. And Winston seemed to fit.'

'So that was the first W?'

'Yes. And after that it just became a bit of a thing.'

'Wilma was originally Alma,' says Richard. 'But I didn't fancy that. Shouting Alma! Alma! was like barking yourself.'

'So we called her Wilma,' says Lolly. 'It was a bit tricky to begin with, because we had to bend the name into shape gradually, so the dog wouldn't get confused.'

'You should've seen her,' says Richard. 'Standing there going AAHHAUUUUWAUUHMMMAAA! Everyone must've thought she was mad.'

'No darling. They thought I was a singer doing vocal exercises.'

I look down at Willard. He returns the gaze.

'So – what about Willard?'

'Ah!' says Lolly. 'Willard was the exception. Willard has always been Willard. Haven't you, darling?'

And I have to admit, I've never seen a dog agree more.

∽

I press the bell and wait. The porch door is shut but the inner one is open, and I can see through into the house. A dark hallway with a baby gate halfway. It's all pretty quiet.

I press the bell again. The button is held together with weathered tape and doesn't look too healthy. It's only then I see there's a piece of paper tacked to the window. The writing has faded almost to nothing but I can just make it out: Bell not working. Please knock.

As soon as I do, there's a wild yapping and snarling from the front room, and a caramel-coloured Jack Russell hurtles out into the hallway and throws herself at the gate. Although 'hurtles' isn't quite right – more a cross between hurtling and a skitterish kind of wobble.

'Peanut! Be quiet! Go in the garden, darling! Go on! In the garden!'

Peanut pays no attention, but spreads her paws, daring me to come any further.

'I'm in here!' says the man.

I put my hand on the handle.

Peanut narrows her eyes and gives a hectic sneeze.

I open the door.

Peanut goes completely nuts. She swells to twice her size, her eyes bulging out, like I've inadvertently cracked the outer door on a space station, and the catastrophic change in pressure is making her pop.

I'm good with dogs but I'm not stupid. I wait for the man to appear, to give me some credibility. Instead I hear him cry out in pain from the front room. There's nothing for it but to go forward and brave the beast.

'No, Peanut!' I say in an Alpha wolf voice. 'No.'

Peanut obviously doesn't care for wolves. As soon as I open the baby gate she goes for me. The only thing that saves me is the fact that Peanut is old and fat and her range of movement is seriously compromised. It also helps that she doesn't have any teeth. All she can manage is a furious gumming of my shoes, which sounds horrendous but is actually quite pleasant, how I imagine it would feel like if I stuck my foot up through the sunroof when I put the car through the car wash. The only real danger is that when I carry on walking she'll trip me up. Maybe that's the plan. Maybe the moment I'm down she'll roll up onto my face and suffocate me. Luckily, I manage to stay upright, though, lifting my legs like some kind of fastidious wading bird, high-stepping through a lake of hostile fish into the front room.

'Good girl!' says the man, approvingly.

Whatever made the man cry out has passed. He's perfectly calm.

'On the sofa, Peanut. On the sofa. Hup!'

The dog is too exhausted from the shoe wars. Anyway, if there was ever a dog in the history of dogs less likely to jump onto a sofa at the word Hup, it's Peanut. She completely ignores the man, choosing instead to wobble exhaustedly over to the far side of the man's chair, collapsing on the carpet with an audible whump like someone delivering coal.

'Oh Peanuuuuut!' says the man, drawing out the last syllable into a tortured wail. Of all the things to despair about, this is the least worst thing. Peanut's obviously used to it. She gives another of her disdainful sneezes, then settles her face onto her paws. With her huge eyes and curled lip, she's a spit for Peter Lorre.

'What are we going to do with you, Peanut?' says the man.

'Does she have a harness?' I ask him.

'There. Behind you,' he says, gesturing to the sofa with his scrubby chin.

I pick it up. It's a complicated affair, heavily-padded corduroy, confusing straps and velcro and snappy fixings. It looks more like a Victorian straitjacket.

I hold it up

'Peanut! Who's a good girl…?'

If the bungalow is quiet when I walk up to the door, it changes the moment I ring the bell. A dog starts barking somewhere deep within the house, and a second later hurls itself against the door, repeatedly impacting the frosted pane like a hairy brown and white football being kicked at the glass.

'Larry! Larry!' says a woman's voice, but the dog only interprets that as an instruction to try harder. He changes tactic and starts trying to rip out the letterbox, presumably to make a hole big enough to squeeze through and reach my throat.

'Just come straight in!' the woman calls. 'He'll be alright.'

It's an act of faith to do it, but Larry's obviously a small dog, and even though I know the smallest dogs have the biggest complexes, I'm reasonably confident I can handle anything he throws at me. Still, mindful of the sharpness of little teeth, I slide the rucksack off my back and hold it low in front of me as I slowly open the door.

'Good boy! There's a good boy!'

Larry backs up, adding a few apoplectic sneezes to his barks, and starts turning wild circles on the spot, like he's winding himself up to helicopter the distance between his jaws and my throat.

Mrs Waring appears round the sitting room door on all fours.

'Oh! Hello!' I say, putting my bag to one side (Larry jumps on it, grabs hold of one of the straps and begins shaking it from side to side, flipping me looks between each thrashing, as if to say: You're next). 'Are you alright?'

'Yes, I'm fine,' she says, in a clipped tone, as if there's absolutely nothing in her behaviour to suggest otherwise.

'Have you fallen? Are you hurt?'

'Not at all,' she says. 'Larry! Will you stop that, please?'

Amazingly, Larry lets go of the bag, looks at Mrs Waring for a moment, then trots over to sniff around my trousers.

'He likes you,' she says. 'That's a start.'

I kneel down on the carpet.

'So tell me how you ended up on the floor,' I say.

'It's very dull,' she says. 'I had another dizzy episode, so I lowered myself down before I fell. I've done it before.'

'Are you in pain?'

'No. Just a little woozy. Now look, could I ask you to do something for me?'

'Of course.'

'It's a bit cheeky, I know, but you see – Larry needs his breakfast and I think that's why he's being such a pest. If he doesn't get his breakfast, he won't leave us alone. So, if you wouldn't mind, could you give him some of the meat that's on the top of the fridge? You'll find a pink bowl on the draining board and a fork with a broken handle. He doesn't need much. His stomach's the size of a mouse.'

Larry has obviously recognised some of the keywords here, because he stops sniffing and sits on his haunches to stare up at me. He's a funny-looking dog, a cross between a Chihuahua and a Jack Russell, with a few chromosomes of Fruit Bat sprinkled on top for interest. He's obviously as elderly as Mrs Waring, a wiry, lopsided sneer to his muzzle, like a grizzled old gunslinger deludedly thinking he can still outdraw anything that rings the bell.

'He'll be in a better mood when he's had some breakfast,' says Mrs Waring.

As if to demonstrate, Larry starts barking again when I stand up to go into the kitchen, and doesn't stop until I've finished scraping some meat out into the bowl.

Meanwhile, Mrs Waring has crawled into the kitchen, too.

'Show me how much you've given him,' she says.

I bend down to show her the bowl.

'Too much,' she says. 'He'll be sick.'

I scrape out a portion and present the bowl to her again, acutely aware that if anyone took a photograph of this scene through the kitchen window, it wouldn't read well in the press. (Broken Britain: Nurse Feeds Elderly Woman Like A Dog).

'Still too much!' she says. 'Lose a third and you might be right.'

I do as she says, and finally get the go-ahead.

Larry clears the bowl in three furious snaps, then starts barking again.

'I don't think it's worked,' I say.

'Nonsense,' says Mrs Waring, turning round to crawl out of the kitchen and into the living room. 'He just doesn't like strangers watching him eat.'

∽ઠ

When I walk into the front garden, a young collie rushes up from the back garden to the rusting, curlicue iron gate that pens it in, pushes its muzzle through the gaps, and barks crazily. I say hello, which only makes it worse, of course. It's a funny-looking dog. The eyes are different colours – one brown, one blue – which, along with the patchwork black and white fur, mismatched paws, one ear up, one ear down, reminds me of an oil painting my Auntie Ollie did of a collie dog, staring up from a hectic, pea-green background.

'Whose dog is that?' I said.

'No-one's,' she said. 'I did it off the calendar.'

All that remains of the keysafe at the front door is the base, though, and I realise that I'm expected to go to the side door, beyond the gate guarded by the mad dog. It gets so excited when it sees me coming back to the gate, it does an insane war dance on its back legs, spinning round on the spot, stopping itself by slamming its paws against the gate, then spinning round in the other direction. It looks pretty crazy, but I think what the hell, and reach in to flip the latch. The dog runs off into the garden, then sprints back with an empty plastic Coke bottle.

'Thanks!' I say.

It drops it at my feet. I toss it away into the garden again, then seize my chance to go through the kitchen door standing open on my right. 'Hell-oooo...'

Maisie is lying on her bed in the gloom. There's a substantial electric mobility scooter in the bedroom doorway – more like one of those big, sit-on mowers – with a seamy jacket slung over the seat and a basket filled with crap strapped to the bumper.

'Over here,' says Maisie.

The dog rushes in behind me and prostrates itself on the floor with the Coke bottle in its mouth, biting it with loud crackles.

'Flash! Leave him alone!' says Maisie. Flash drops the bottle and smile-pants up at me. I stroke Flash's head, then straighten up, breathe in, and squeeze past the scooter into the bedroom.

'The diet starts tomorrow,' I say.

I'm guessing there's been a partial deep clean at some point. There are lots of yellow bags zip-locked, piled up around the place. Maisie's bed seems enormous, Maisie spread-eagled on it, like a depressed housewife cast adrift in a yellow ocean on a giant orange sponge.

''Scuse the mess,' she says.

The phone rings. She grunts and rolls towards the side table. Before I have a chance to pass the phone to her, she knocks it off its base and the two things fall down the back of the bed. To be fair, it would be difficult NOT to knock anything off Maisie's side table. It's a cheap, warped affair, made worse by the fact it's littered with stuff – bottles of spray, a glass of water, a mobile phone, an alarm clock. When I retrieve the phone and the base, hand Maisie the phone, and put the base back on the stand, I knock the alarm clock off. When I retrieve the alarm clock and set it down again, I knock the phone base back onto the floor.

'Jesus Christ!' I say.

'Whoopsie!' says Maisie. She holds the phone to her nose and prods the buttons myopically. 'Dunno who that was,' she says after a while. She hands me the phone. 'Don't drop it,' she says.

I rearrange the side table as best I can, then start in on the examination.

Turns out, the phone call was from the pharmacist. She rings again and this time Maisie manages to answer it without anything else happening. There's a long conversation, Maisie saying yes or no or yes or no or sometimes, all in a bored, non-committal way – then hands the phone to me.

'She wants to talk to you,' she says.

The pharmacist is someone I know well. She has the kind of

incisive questioning that's light and pleasant but still makes you sit up a little straighter.

'Maisie says she hasn't got her medication. It should be in a green bag somewhere. Could you check for me?'

I don't have to check very hard; the bag is right there in front of me, beside the table. Not only that, the drug chart in the folder at the foot of the bed shows that the carers gave the morning dose as prescribed.

'Good!' says the pharmacist. 'That's a relief! Although why she told me she didn't have it... is she confused this morning?'

'No, she seems pretty orientated and okay. All her obs are fine...'

Flash has climbed on the bed by this point. He's lying on his back with his legs in the air as Maisie tickles his tummy.

'Who's a silly boy? Who's a silly boy?'

Flash stares at me with his tongue hanging out, his mismatched eyes spinning with ecstasy.

'She seems fine,' I say.

The pharmacist has arranged to visit later to check up on things. I say goodbye to Maisie, and with the dog leaping around me like a species of giant flea, I see myself out, closing the gate as quietly as I can behind me.

I open my laptop and write my notes in the car. There are a few things to sort out, so I'm there fifteen minutes or so. I'm just about to finish up and move on when I hear a clatter from the gate. Maisie is coming out on the electric scooter, Flash trotting by her side. Maisie pauses at the front of the garden. She pulls out a packet of fags, nips one out with her lips, lights the fag with a flip of her Zippo, puts the packet back in her pocket, all in one smooth, practised motion. Then she sits there smoking a minute or two, looking right and left along the street, blowing smoke from her nose in a business-like way. Then she twists the key on the scooter again and heads right, at speed, to the park, I'd guess, with Flash high-stepping alongside her, trying to avoid the wheels. On the top of the basket, I can see an empty plastic Coke bottle rattling from side to side.

I wonder who put it there.

⤚

I've never seen such an old stair lift. It sits at the bottom of the stairs like a traction engine whose wheels have fallen off. It even has a hatch under the seat, which must be where the coal goes.

'It was my husband's,' says Maria. 'Shame it's broken. It means I can't go upstairs.'

'What about getting it fixed?'

She shakes her head.

'The company went bust years ago.'

'But surely someone somewhere would know what to do with it?'

'I know exactly what to do with it. Throw it in a skip and start again. But I'm alright downstairs. I've got everything I need.'

I follow her into the living room, almost tripping over a metal milk holder with three pints in it that Maria has brought inside and put in the doorway.

'Shall I put these in the fridge?'

'Yes. Sorry, dear. That's as far as I got.'

Maria was discharged from the hospital after treatment for a chest infection, referred to us for ongoing care.

'I do alright,' she says, when I bring her through some tea. 'I'm not as badly off as others. I've got two gay gentlemen living next door. They're so lovely and kind. They do my shopping and what have you. Most mornings they knock on the door when they take the dog out. They've got this little dog, you see. Don't ask me what sort it is. I'm not good with dogs. I pretend to be interested but between you and me it's not that impressive. Its fur sticks out all over the place and it has this odd, cross-eyed look, like someone clonked it with a frying pan. I wouldn't trust it as far as I could throw it, but they seem to like it, which is the main thing.'

We chat as I check her over. She tells me about her husband, Jack.

A small businessman with a big laugh, apparently.

'Yes,' she says. 'It's true. I married the boss. That's him, there…'

She points to a photo in a frame: An elderly man sitting in a chair, Maria standing behind him with her arms around his shoulders, the point of her chin on the top of his head. The picture has stood in direct sunlight for so long the colour has faded. All the flesh tones have merged, leaving a blurry but strangely transcendent quality to their faces. Only the stronger patterns remain: the curve of Jack's glasses, Maria's auburn curls, the laces on Jack's shoes.

'I still miss him, all these years later,' she says, carefully taking a sip of tea. 'Maybe I should get a cat. What d'you think?'

2: Cats

Supermarket orchids: a conspiracy theorist's dream. You seem them everywhere, the arching, fleshy leaves, the elongated stalks, indestructible, scarcely needing soil, let alone water, silently keeping an eye on things from a million kitchen windowsills. The only plant on earth with a chance of survival in Stanley's flat.

So it's a measure of the place that even the supermarket orchids have died.

In their defence, though, you would have to think that a supermarket orchid would face better odds being given as a farewell present to an astronaut, spending years in space, and then being set out on a rock on the surface of Mars to make it more homey, than on a shelf in Stanley's flat.

It's not for want of trying. He has lots of plants dotted around the place – the remains, at least. Nothing survives. It's even a challenge identifying the original plant from the scattering of papery stalks and the random pots of desiccated fronds.

There's a shelf of dead plants above the washing machine in the utility room. On top of the washing machine is a hefty ginger cat, one paw draped lovingly over the front of the door as the machine rattles and judders in a manic spin cycle.

'There's nothing Rastus likes better than sleeping on the washing machine,' says Stanley. 'I think he thinks it's a big mummy cat.'

'With one hell of a purr.'

'Is that it, Rastus? Do you think the machine's purring?'

If Rastus hears us (or is, in fact, alive), he makes no sign.

We both look at him there for a while, then Stanley tuts, and leads me further down the hall.

'Make yourself at home!' he says, gesturing to a living room of dead plants.

There's another enormous, and enormously furry cat, draped over a brightly-coloured, leather Moroccan pouffe.

'His name's Bartlefink,' says Stanley.

'Like the film?'

'There's a film?'

'Oh – no – that's Barton Fink.'

'Hmm.'

'Great name, anyway. Where did you get it?'

He shrugs.

'I don't know. He just looked like one.'

I try to think what he means. If I think of the name Bartlefink, I think of a comic book detective in a raincoat and hat, although I don't think I've ever seen anything like that, so I'm not sure why. To me, this huge, bouffant cat, blessed with the kind of flat and cross-eyed expression you might see on a creature who'd turned to look at you in the street and walked into a lamppost – if anything, at a push, I'd have called it Monstro. And I like cats.

'He's got such a sweet temper,' says Stanley, bending down with an audible crack like his legs don't articulate at the knee so much as break in the middle. 'C'mon Bartlefink! C'mon!'

Whether it's me, or he's normally this contemptuous, it's hard to tell. But after staring at me a good long while, and then giving one of his paws a peremptory shake in the manner of a street hoodlum who'd shank me for a packet of Dreamies, he about-tails and stomps off into the kitchen.

'He'll be in later, you'll see,' says Stanley, using me as a counter-balance to straighten up again.

I don't know, though. The noise of that cat flap sounds pretty final to me.

✍

'Sometimes I think it would be nice to have an animal. A cat, you know. Some company. But you're not allowed animals in the block. I can understand why, of course. There are quite a few people here. If everyone had an animal, what on earth would it be like? A zoo, probably. Whipsnade Zoo!'

'I don't do so bad, though. I don't bother with the idiot box much. I have all these books, you see. When I was working, I don't think I ever read. Too busy travelling around, keeping the business afloat. To the Outer Hebrides, on one occasion. Sounds like a long way – and it was – but it was worth it. I think. Now, the furthest I manage is from the bedroom to the kitchen. Although sometimes, if the weather's nice like today, I'll drag these sorry old bones out into the front garden. There's a little bench there, under the roses. I'll take a book and sit there, and read, or just watch the world go by.'

'The odd cat.'

Buddy Holly is sprawled on the back of the sofa, Eddie Cochrane is staring down at me from the top of the wardrobe, and Elvis Presley is lying on the floor with his paws in the air, waiting to be tickled.

'That's so Elvis,' I tell Pat, leaning in.

'He's still quite kittenish,' she says. 'You wouldn't think he was twelve.'

Elvis grabs my hand with his front paws and rakes me with his back, but keeps his claws retracted. His mouth gapes, his eyes deepen to perfect circles of black, and his ears flatten.

'He loves that,' says Pat.

'He totally looks like Elvis,' I tell her. 'Maybe in his cape years.'

'I thought about making him a cape once,' she says. 'But I didn't want him swallowing the rhinestones.'

'Okay. Enough now, Elvis. What about you, Pat? How are you feeling today?'

'Oh I'm alright,' says Pat. 'I'm always alright. I don't know what all the fuss is about.'

'I think it was because you fainted and broke your hip.'

'Yes, but – these things happen.'

'Do they know why you fainted?'

'I got up too quickly. Eddie and Buddy were fighting and I had to sort them out. Next thing I knew I was staring up at them, and when I tried to get up my hip was agony.'

'Did you have a carelink button then?'

'No! It's only since. No – I had to crawl to the phone. It was only on the hall table but it may as well have been on the moon. Luckily Ian across the way has a key, so the ambulance didn't have to break the door down.'

'That's something anyway.'

'I was in hospital for ages. It was torture. My poor cats. I was worried sick.'

'Did Ian look after them?'

'No. He's allergic. If he sees a cat on the telly he sneezes. No – they had to go to a cat hotel, out in the country.'

'Sounds lovely.'

'It wasn't. It cost me an arm and a leg. And I don't know what they spend the money on because it certainly isn't food. They were half starved when I got them back.'

I can't imagine any of these cats half-starved. I struggle to imagine how Eddie Cochrane makes it up to the top of the wardrobe without a hoist.

I run through the usual observations, blood pressure, temperature, SATS and the rest. Everything checks out. Pat's blood pressure drops a little when she stands, but not precipitously, and ever since the accident she knows to do things slowly, in stages.

'I'm guessing you like rock and roll then,' I say, taking the pressure cuff off her arm and nodding in the direction of Buddy Holly, who's sitting staring at me from the kitchen with such a fixed expression on his face I feel unaccountably possessed by the urge to walk over and open a tin.

'Not particularly,' says Pat. 'I got them all as kittens, and they were so funny, I could just see them jumping around on stage, playing guitar.'

❧

Mac is sitting on the balcony, smoking a cigar. It's so bright when I step out to join him, I can barely open my eyes.

'What a view!' I say, sitting down on one of the wicker seats opposite.

'I've missed it so much,' he says. 'I was going a little crazy back in that hospital.'

I'm not kidding about the view. The balcony overlooks a busy port area, stacks of lumber, pyramids of gravel, warehouses, through-ways, the deep waters of the quayside in contrast to the silvery-grey ocean on the other side. It's eerily quiet, though. All the cranes and forklifts are parked up. No people, no ships. Even the seagulls look uneasy, gliding past, wondering where the change is, what it means.

I've been asked to find out what Mac needs immediately, with the longer-term palliative teams to follow. I was a little nervous coming to see him. It's never clear from the documentation just exactly what the patient knows or has accepted about their diagnosis. You have to tread carefully, feeling-out the right approach. Mac makes it easy, though. From the outset he's able to talk freely about the treatment options that gradually closed off to him, the hard decisions, the plan as it currently stands.

'I don't need anything for the minute,' he says, blowing out another, luxurious cloud of smoke. 'I'm getting by, taking it as it comes. I know it's going to get harder but for the minute I'm alright.'

I tell him how the service works, how quickly we can get back in touch if anything changes.

'We're just on the end of the phone,' I say. 'A couple of hours and we're back.'

'That's good to know,' he says.

His family join us. We sit in a semicircle, squinting out over the silent dockyard.

'They asked me whether I wanted to go to the hospice,' he says. 'But – n'ah! I'm not there yet. Maybe it'll come, maybe it won't. I'm not sure.'

'You could stay at home, if you wanted,' I tell him. 'We'd have to change things round a little, nearer the time. Put in a hospital bed. Other stuff. It's up to you. It's so lovely here. And you'd have the nursing teams coming in to support you.'

'Everyone's been so good,' he says.

'But the hospice is always an option, too.'

'I mean – it's a nice place and everything,' he says, leaning forwards and carefully knocking the ash from his cigar against the edge of the ashtray. 'I went there for a bit a little while ago.'

'What did you think?'

'They even had a cat wandering about the place. The way they treated him, you'd think he was one of the consultants.'

'Yeah! I've seen that cat! He's hilarious!'

'If you like cats. Which I do. No – I've got nothing against the place. But it's just – I don't know. You get chatting to the geezer in the next bed, and it's always at the back of your mind that they're dying. And the guy opposite. And the guy next to you. Stuff like that. It can really freak you out.'

He takes another toke on the cigar. A lone seagull wheels and turns overhead. And in the near distance, and further away, the waters around the dock, the sea running out to the horizon, every last plane and detail of it – everything – crackles and jumps with light.

Gary's shown hostility to health care professionals in the past, and the record says we're only to visit in pairs. I'm a little early meeting up with Lisa, so I park up outside and take the opportunity to finish off some notes on the laptop. I've just settled in to start writing when Gary's door opens and a woman steps out. She's tall and pale and pinched-looking, wearing a green and black nylon tracksuit, her long hair dragged back in a ponytail. She takes out a fag packet and is just about to have a smoke when she sees me, sitting there. I wind down the window to tell her I've come to see Gary and I'm just waiting on my colleague, but before I can say anything she shoves the fags back in her pocket, walks backwards into the doorway, and maintaining eye contact for as long as she can, slowly shuts the door.

It doesn't augur well.

Lisa turns up ten minutes later. I'd trust any of the team to go on a difficult visit, but if I had to choose, Lisa would be it. The Italians have a word for how she is: sprezzatura – a kind of nonchalance or ease, wearing her skill lightly, with great warmth and humanity, as if it's really nothing and no trouble at all, and what was it that needed doing, now, and suddenly it's done, and everyone feels better.

'How's it going there, Jim?' she says, padding along the street. 'Have you been waitin' long?'

We go together through the terrible little garden, knock and wait. There are sounds from inside. An exchange of light and shadow in the frosted panes above the door. A clattering of the lock, and suddenly the door opens.

A bare-chested man, his eyes squeezed shut, his smile as wide and flat as the Man in the Moon.

'I expect you're wondering why I'm half naked?' he says. 'Only I was just having a carton of cherry and raspberry squash, and I didn't want to get any on my t-shirt.'

'No. That would stain, right enough,' says Lisa.

'Yes,' he says. 'You'd never get it out.'

There's a steep, bare board staircase just behind the man. The woman I saw earlier is crouched at the top, peering down at us on all fours.

'Don't listen to him!' she shouts. 'He sees ghosts!'

'Okay, now! That's interesting!' says Lisa. 'So… is yer man through in this room, or …'

'Ye-es,' says the man, stepping to one side and knocking on the door. 'I say Gary? There are two lovely nurses to see you.'

'Show them in but keep Jackie out.'

'Righto.'

The man pushes the door open and nods for us to go through. Meanwhile, Jackie has started coming down the stairs, slowly feeling with her feet for each tread whilst her face stays as fixed on us as a steadicam.

'Now, now, Jacqueline!' says the man. 'Gary doesn't want you there.'

Jackie gives a petulant scream, sits down on the step and folds her arms.

'After you,' says the man.

We step into the room.

It's hot as a sauna – the foetid, barrelling kind, where you fling urine on the coals instead of water. I wonder how long Gary's been lying on his bed like this, his teeth grey and claggy as if he's been snacking on ash. It's like we've stumbled into a mausoleum, where the occupant took up early residency for want of anything better to do, and his stuff got chucked in after him. There are two posters on the wall: Jimi Hendricks leaning back from a guitar solo; The Beatles all in a line.

'Wha'd'ya want?' says Gary.

'Hello there!' says Lisa, offering him her hand. 'Nice to meet you, Gary. This is my colleague Jim. We've been asked to come and see how you're doing.'

'How'm I doing?' he says. 'I'm NOT doing.'

'What's troubling you today, then, Gary?'

'I can't keep nothin' down. I feel sick all the time. I've got no energy. I'm wracked with pain. Is that enough for you?'

'That's enough for anyone,' she says. 'You poor thing. Let's see what's what, then. I'll just do your blood pressure and whatnot and see how that is, and Jim here'll take a wee bit o'blood, if that's okay?'

'I don't care,' he says. 'You may as well. I've got to go to the toilet first, though.'

He nods in the direction of a commode whose pot has been removed so it can fit over a bucket.

'Do you need a hand getting out of bed, there, Gary?' says Lisa.

'I'll be alright, thanks,' he says. 'If you wouldn't mind stepping outside for a bit.'

'No worries.'

We leave him to it.

Out in the hall the bare-chested man has gone and Jackie is nowhere to be seen. Instead, an ancient black and white cat yowls as it approaches us from the living room. I'm guessing it's blind because both its eyes are white. It feels its way along the wall, one paw at a time. I crouch down and hold my hand out. The cat stops, sniffs the air, then moves in my direction. When it gets closer, I see that its tongue pokes out to the side, too.

'Poor wee fella!' says Lisa.

I stroke the cat. It starts purring – a deep, rumbly sound – his tail pointing straight up, as if he's absorbing the affection and transmitting it somewhere.

'The cat! The cat knows everything!' says a voice at the top of the stairs.

Jackie is there, staring down at us again.

'Oh – they do, though, don't they?' says Lisa, smiling up at her. 'Cats. You're right there, Jackie. They certainly do.'

Magda bangs the horn with the heel of her hand, the force of it pushing her back into the seat.

'Fucking hell! Would it kill you to indicate? How we supposed to know what you going to do at roundabout? What do you think I am? Fucking mind-reader?'

She drives on.

'My father used to be traffic cop. He made it big thing to learn. He say to me "It doesn't matter if it's one, two, three o'clock in morning and no-one on road for miles. You make manoeuvre, you indicate. Because this way it becomes automatic habit, and you do it whenever you drive, without thinking."'

She's forced to give way to an oncoming car.

'Jesus fucking bastard! Sorry – I know is bad to swear. But please!

Where these people learn to drive? Fucking CLOWN school?'

One of our carers has gone sick, so I've been asked to help Magda out with a double-up call. It's to Rita, a very elderly and frail woman who has deteriorated significantly in the last few days. The regular care company don't have capacity to pick up the increased calls yet, so we've stepped in to bridge the gap.

'Rita is lovely woman,' says Magda, pushing her enormous sunglasses up into her bleach blonde hair. 'But then you see, I only do lovely womans.'

She jabs at the keysafe with one hand and retrieves the keys without even seeming to look, everything so slickly done it's like watching a stage magician.

'Rita has lovely cat,' she says, opening the door. 'But she is grumpy in morning, like you. Helllloooooo? Rita? It's the carers, darling. Good morning. We're coming up there…'

I follow her up the stairs into a large, dimly-lit sitting room with a hospital bed at one end. Rita is lying in the bed, surrounded by cushions and bolsters, the mattress raised in the middle to crook her legs up. She turns her head to the side to smile at us, the skin beneath her chin spare and slack, her whole body giving the impression of a generalised falling away, as if life was a tidal force leaving her now, declining with the last phase of the moon.

Almost immediately there's an imperious yowling sound, and an enormous black cat stomps into the room behind us. The cat is wearing an expression so furious you could simply draw an X with a marker pen and be done. She advances into the middle of the carpet, sits on her haunches with an audible plump, licks her lips once, and waits.

'Here is cat!' says Magda, to avoid any confusion. 'I'm sorry, I forgot already. What is cat called?' she says to Rita, who manages to say without any interruption to her smile that the cat is called Juniper.

'Juniper? Huh. I thought was Jupiter. Juniper? Like berry? Is this what you call it, berry?'

I nod.

'They use it to make gin,' I say. 'I think that's where the name comes from.'

'Juniper?'

'I think gin is short for ginevere or something. Dutch maybe. Which means juniper.'

'Huh.'

She turns to Rita.

'You like gin, Rita? Is that why you name your cat Juniper? Maybe you have other cat called vodka?'

Rita closes her eyes and shakes her head imperceptibly.

'No worry,' says Magda. 'Let us sort you out, darling...'

After Rita is freshened up, the sheets changed and everything taken care of, Magda plays with the cat whilst I write up the notes. Magda knows where Juniper's toys are kept; straightaway she fetches a small plastic fishing rod with a crinkly bee on the end of a string and dandles it in the air above Juniper's head. Juniper swats at it – a little half-heartedly, it seems to me, flashing me looks now and again as if to say: Look – I've just got to attend to this damned bee business and I'll be with you directly.

'What is matter with you today, cat?' says Magda. 'Is my friend here distracting you? Is that what it is? Hmm?' She gives up, tosses the rod on the sofa, and subjects Juniper to one more colossal stroke of the head and neck – so vigorously that as a matter of survival, Juniper has to stand and brace herself with her front paws, raising her tail straight up in the air to deflect the energy into the ceiling.

Magda picks up her bag to go.

'I love this funny cat, Rita,' she says. 'We have cat back home, Puszek. But he is farm cat. Like baby tiger, you know? Puszek is so big now he drive the tractor.'

Rita bats a skeletal hand in the air.

'Okay, darling,' says Magda, taking Rita's hand and squeezing it. 'You take care now. We see you later. Okay? Okay. And don't worry. We put key back in key safe.'

Juniper jumps up onto the bed, and immediately begins paddling on the duvet with its paws.

'Good girl,' says Magda. 'That's it!'

❦

Rosie is more confused than usual, according to Rosie – the other Rosie, I mean, the one who lives at the end of the road and comes in most days to help. The fact that her husband Jim has the same name as me, only adds to the confusion. He's amiable enough, placid as an old turtle who swapped his shell for a corduroy jacket. If Rosie Two hadn't introduced him as her husband, I'd think he'd tagged along by mistake. When she asks him to fetch in Rosie One's address book from the kitchen, he wanders back in, flicking through a photo album.

'Look at you in front of the Sphinx, Rosie!' he says. 'Well, well.'

'Oh for heaven's sake,' says Rosie Two, and goes to get the address book herself.

Rosie One is sitting in her armchair, held in place by an enormous, ash-grey cat. The cat stares at me, its head bobbing up and down and its eyes pulled wide in time with the vigorous strokes.

'Poor Jonesie!' says Rosie One. 'I fell on him, you know. Squashed him flat! Broke my fall, though, didn't you, Jonesie? Hey? You broke mummy's fall, didn't you? You clever thing!'

'Tripped you up, more like,' says Rosie Two, striding back in from the kitchen and handing me the address book. 'That cat. It's an absolute monster. Anyway. There! Karen's number. The next of kin. Apparently.'

Jim Two has drifted over to the bookcase, tutting and exclaiming as he makes his way along the shelves with his head crooked so far to one side his ear is practically on his shoulder.

'Well, well!' he says, carefully sliding a book out. 'Who'd have thought!'

'Jim!' says Rosie Two. 'You're supposed to be making breakfast!'

'Am I? Oh, right,' he says. 'Absolutely. Of course. Breakfast. Yes.'

And he wanders away in the opposite direction to the kitchen with a book in his hand. Rosie Two goes after him.

'Nothing's the same since my darling husband died,' says Rosie One.

She's looking at a portrait on the sideboard, a broad-faced, smiling man in a white naval uniform.

'I'm sorry,' I say. 'What was his name?'

'Jim.'

'Jim? Not another one!'

'Well,' she says, turning back to me. 'My Jim was the first.'

'So – how did you come to fall?'

'I was going in to my mindfulness class when I tripped on the step.'

Myrna is an engaging patient. Seventy-three going on seventeen, hair silvery blue and woven in plaits; tie-dye dress, yellow and black stockings, moccasins. Above her, hanging from the paper moon lampshade, a dreamcatcher.

A large, tortoiseshell-and-white cat struts in through the living room door into the middle of the carpet, its tail straight up, just the very tip of it flexing languorously left and right and left again.

'Pippin!' says Myrna, holding out her hands. 'Where've you been, you naughty boy?'

Pippin wanders towards me for a closer inspection, cautiously sniffing the hem of my trousers.

'Extraordinary!' says Myrna, clasping her hands together. 'He's never done that before.'

'We've got a cat,' I say.

'I don't know,' says Myrna. 'I don't know. He's a rescue. He's had bad experiences. There's something else...'

Now that Pippin has our full attention he decides to put on a display. He walks round and round on the carpet between us, eventually collapsing to one side. Then he arches his back and stretches his legs, almost doubling in size. After holding that position for a moment or two, his ears go back, his eyes darken, and he suddenly starts clawing the carpet, hauling himself in a mad circle, which ends up with one back leg in the air and his nose stuffed under his tail to give himself a clean.

'We're making such progress!' says Myrna.

Around her on the sofa are piles of red wool and a stack of knitted red squares. Myrna reaches over and picks one up.

'Cat jackets,' she says, giving it a gentle shake. 'You know – jackets. For cats. When the weather's bad.'

'They're lovely.'

'I donate them to an animal welfare shop. I used to work there, but the stories upset me too much and I had to come away. I like to do what I can, though.'

She holds the half-finished jacket up.

'I might trim it with a little fur, to make it more Christmassy. Mind you, I don't really celebrate Christmas. When you think of all those turkeys and what they do to them. It just makes you... it makes you...'

She looks tearful. But then Pippin jumps up beside her.

'Pippin!' she says, putting her knitting down again and leaning forwards so they can rub heads. 'What a truly magical little cat you are!'

3: Stars in Battledress

If you hadn't guessed from the wall-mounted displays of cap badges, ribbons and medals, the fading photographs of men on parade, smoking in hospital beds or raising tin cups sitting on the sides of a tank, from the shelves filled with books on the Second World War to the cabinets ornamented with polished anti-tank shells, riding crops and the like – well, then, you'd probably still guess Mr Bradford was an old soldier by the way he sat in the chair, hands draped over his walking stick, feet planted shoulder width, back straight, his two bruised eyes glittering.

'Tell me again who you are, please, and what you have come to do,' he says.

Mr Bradford has been referred to us by the hospital. The story was that he'd gone to catch another elderly resident as she fell backwards in the garden, putting himself between her and some plant pots, the geriatric equivalent of taking a bullet. He was lucky not to break anything ('...but then I always was quite lucky in that regard,' he says). What the episode has highlighted, though, is Mr Bradford's growing frailty. He's been struggling to cope at home, too proud to ask for help, gradually drifting in terms of personal hygiene, nutrition and so on. The good news is there are lots of practical things we can do to help, and Mr Bradford is happy to accept.

'You'll appreciate this story, being a military man,' I say to him, taking a pause and resting on my laptop.

'Go on,' he says. There's a sudden chill in the room, as if he'd turned the angle-poise light into my face and slowly lit a cigarette.

'Where I grew up, in Wisbech. Cambridgeshire. The Fens...'

'I know where it is,' he says.

'Well... the guy who ran the local electrical repair shop – this very unassuming man, little round spectacles, bald head – used to fix the Hoovers and radios and whatnot...'

'Ye-es,' says Mr Bradford.

'Well...his name was Mr Cox.'

'Mr Cox?'

'Yes. Anyway, all these years we just knew him as Mr Cox, the guy who fixed your radio and where you could buy those little pifco torches, you know? The red square ones with the big slidey white switches...'

'Tell me about Mr Cox,' says Mr Bradford.

'Well... turns out he was a war hero.'

'A war hero?'

'Yes. Have you heard of the Bruneval Raid? When a team of paratroopers went over to France to dismantle a radar station?'

'I know what the Bruneval Raid is.'

'Well... Mr Cox was the technician who went with them. To dismantle it. Even though it was packed full of Germans. I mean – it was quite a daring thing.'

'Yes. The Bruneval Raid,' says Mr Bradford, picking an invisible piece of lint from his threadbare trousers, dropping it off to the side, and then slowly directing his attention back to me. 'The only operation successfully led by a parachute battalion, I believe.'

Leslie opens the door, mid-chuckle, like he was waiting there all this time to do just that.

'Well come in! Come in!' he laughs. 'We don't stand on ceremony here you know!'

I hold the door so he can let go, grabbing him when he almost plunges backwards into an umbrella stand, then holding onto him till he finds his balance again. 'Thanking you,' he says. 'Must take more water with it. Er-hem. This way!' He walks ahead, rocking from side to side, lifting his legs stiffly from the hip and working his arms, like a robot in an old sci-fi movie.

'Through here!' he says, as if there was anywhere else to go in the tiny flat, leading me into a sitting room with two armchairs conspicuously together in front of the television, one of them now being used as a place to put magazines and letters. 'Sit where you like!' he says. ''scuse the mess.'

Leslie's doing well for ninety-eight. The only time his bright mood slips is when he mentions his wife, who died a couple of years ago. 'We were a good team,' he says. 'I miss her a lot. It doesn't seem fair. Still – that's the way of the world! I'll see her again soon.'

The doctor referred Leslie in to us for physio and nursing care, nothing too drastic. He's pretty independent. Goes out most days – or did, before his fall. He has a son who lives a couple of miles away. Visits all the time.

'My confidence got dented along with my pride' Leslie says, squeezing his eyes together as he wipes his round glasses on his untucked shirt. 'Still – I'll find it again, don't you worry! You can't keep old chaps like me down for long!' He puts his glasses back on and blinks at me happily. There you are! I can see who I'm dealing with now!'

When I'm done and writing up my notes, Leslie hands me a paperback he's been reading – a history of the spitfire.

'Any good?' I say, flipping it over to read the blurb.

'It's alright,' he says. 'My son got it for me. I was a bit disappointed, to be honest with you. It doesn't mention my lot at all.'

'Oh yeah? Who was that?'

'The One Five Two. Black Panthers. So called 'cos we had a panther on the side, jumping over the roundel. I was one of the technicians, loading 'em up, fixing 'em when they went wrong – well, trying to, at least. Out in Burma.'

'That must've been tough.'

'We got through it. I remember one of the new pilots, South African he was. Tall, handsome chap. Big dimple in his chin, like Superman. He says to me one day, he says Sorry to trouble you old chap, but would you be able to do anything with this blasted watch? And he handed it over, and it was this big ol' German thing, big as my head. Beautiful it was, a real precision piece. Lord only knows how he got it. Or how he lifted his arm when it was on. Anyway, he says to me he says The blasted thing's losing time but it's my lucky watch and I don't want to fly without it. So I looked it over, but honestly I didn't have the foggiest. I mean – half the time with dodgy instruments you just chucked 'em out and replaced 'em. Why they ever made me a technician in the first place is a mystery. So anyway, I give it back to him and I said Sorry squire! I think you'll have to get it fixed in Berlin next time you're over. So he took it back, and they flew out on a mission that night, and he never came back. And I think about that watch sometimes. I think if I'd have took it from him to fix, I'd probably still have it now. Not so lucky after all, was it?'

'That's quite a story.'

'Don't get me started,' he laughs. 'Change the record, that's what Vera used to say.'

He seems to dip a little.

I tell him about Mr Burton, the guy who ran the corner sweet shop we used to go to on our way back from school.

'He was this huge guy, big shining face, hardly any teeth, in a shopcoat with all the buttons straining and scuff marks down the front where he wiped the sugar off his hands. And he used to stand at the counter with all these sweet jars behind him, rows and rows of them, breathing hard whilst we made our choice. Sherbet lemons, gobstoppers, aniseed balls, flying saucers – you name it. And whenever he weighed the sweets out from the jars, he'd pop one in his mouth. It was like: A quarter for you and one for me. A quarter for you and one for me. It was only years later I found out he was on the Burma railway. Just skin and bone when he got liberated.'

'He was lucky to get out of that one,' says Leslie. 'Poor chap. It was a hard business, that's for sure. He was probably just making up for lost time. Anyway – how'm I looking? A-one? Or a ticket home?'

And he gives his knees a vigorous rub, like he's priming an engine or something, winding himself up, ready for action.

'But dash it all! We haven't even been introduced!'

I shake Ken's hand, for the fifth time.

'I'm Jim. From the hospital. How d'you do?'

'Jim, you say?'

'Yes.'

'Welcome, Jim!'

'Thank you!'

'Now – Jim. Can you tell me something?'

'Of course.'

'Why am I here?'

'Well – this is your home, Ken.'

'Yes – but why am I here?'

'This is the best place to look after you.'

'If you say so,' he says, leaning back in the chair, suddenly unimpressed with the whole affair.

He watches me unpack my kit.

'What are you proposing to do now?' he says.

'Take your blood pressure and temperature and what have you. If that's okay.'

'Be my guest!' he says, waving a hand in the air. 'It's all the same to me.'

'Thanks!'

His live-in carer Yasmina comes in with a tray of tea.

'You want different war film on, Ken?'

'Do what, y'say?'

It's Where Eagles Dare, the bit where Clint Eastwood knocks on the door of the radio room, says hello and then shoots everyone. The TV's up loud anyway, but with the machine gun and the AAAIIIIGH screams, I'm wincing and flinching as much as Clint.

'Some war film different to this one,' shouts Yasmina, going over to switch it off. 'You've seen this one too many time, Ken. Too many time. All the Germans they are killt by now.'

The way she says killt – emphasised by the severely sculpted lines of her makeup.

'As you wish,' he says.

'Look. I have new one for you, Ken. World at War, Ken. You like World at War?'

'Spoiler alert. We win!' I say.

'What means, we win?' says Yasmina, kneeling down to operate the DVD player, poking one finger through the hole, drawing Where Eagles Dare out and wearing it on her finger like a donut, switching it with the other, jolting the DVD tray back into place, hitting the right sequence of buttons on the control, all in one fluid movement.

'The war. We won the war.'

'Which?'

'I don't know. Either. Both. I think.'

'Oh. This is good news.'

She turns to Ken.

'Ken! We won war!'

He frowns at her, then at me, and then smiling, reaches out his hand.

'But dash it all! We haven't even been introduced!'

The sepulchral tones of the World at War theme tune begin to play.

'Great,' says Yasmina, standing up and brushing the front of her uniform down. 'Now I have this song in my head all day.'

'Shall I take my shoes off?'

'Oh no!' says Rita. 'This is a real home – not a show home!'

I'm conscious that my shoes are sopping wet, though, so I slip them off anyway.

'I do it at home,' I say. 'I'd feel bad otherwise.'

'This is a real home, not a show home!' she says, repeating herself – whether because it's a catchphrase of hers, or because she likes the sound of it, I'm not sure.

'Follow me!' she says, and leads me through the house.

It certainly has the feel of a show home. Or even a gallery, given the number of paintings of stags on snowy crags and jugged hares lying among bunches of grapes, all in heavy gilt frames. Ernest, Rita's husband, sits in a chair at the far end of the house, like a decrepit attendant who dozed through his lunch break and on into his nineties.

'Darling? There's a nurse to see you!' says Rita. She waves me over to him, then lowers herself very correctly, debutante-style, into a Louis Quinze chair, her legs angled to the right, her hands folded in her lap.

'What happened to your shoes?' says Ernie, peering at me over his glasses.

'They were soaking wet. I didn't want to make a mess on your carpet.'

'I said to him, darling,' says Rita. 'I said to him: This is a real home. Not a show home!'

'Hear that?' he says. 'So now you know.'

All Ernest's observations are within normal range – his blood pressure, temperature, heart rate and so on.

'What were you expecting?' he says. 'I'm perfectly fine. It's this damned back.'

'Let the gentleman do his job, darling,' says Rita, absentmindedly playing with her wedding ring, slipping it off, then on, then off again. 'He used to be a sniper, you know. In the war, of course,' she adds, hurriedly, to clear up any misunderstanding.

'A sniper?'

'What of it?' he snaps.

'No. Nothing. It sounds fascinating.'

'Hmm,' he says, and watches me closely as I fill out his obs chart. To cover the silence – and to find out more about his sniper years – I dig deep for some personal story I could use.

'I had a go at skeet shooting once,' I say. 'It was a work's outing. I really liked it.'

'Skeet shooting?'

'Yes. Clay pigeons.'

'I know what skeet shooting is.'

'It was really good! That bit where they chuck the clays along the ground, and they bounce around all over the place. That was fun. You know. Picking them off.'

'Fun?' says Ernest, horrified. 'Fun? If by fun you mean waving your weapon around like a lunatic, blasting in the general direction of where you think something's going to end up, well, then, perhaps. But I'm not talking about some random spread of pellets. I'm talking about the precise placing of a single, large calibre bullet. I'm talking about controlling one's breathing, slowing one's pulse. Taking a clean shot.'

And he glares at me over his glasses again, eyebrows quivering, drawing a bead.

'It's my second marriage,' says Rita. 'Would you like a cup of tea?'

Mr Curtis' maisonette flat is so high up, on an unadopted dirt road close to the cliff edge, he could rent it out to the coast guard as a lookout. When he tells me he used to be a submariner, it's hard not to think he had so many years being underwater he wanted to live the rest of his life as high above the surface as he could get.

'So what did you do on the submarines?' I ask him, unwrapping the blood pressure cuff with a rasp of velcro.

'I was a spy,' he says, rubbing his arm.'

'A spy? I didn't know they had spies on submarines.'

I imagine a guy in breathing apparatus, shadowing his goggles as he peers through a porthole.

'Radio operators, you know. Specialists. We used to sit on the sea bed for weeks on end, monitoring the Russians coming and going. We had to wear slippers and creep about. We had no idea where we were. Could've been under the Arctic. Could've been the Bahamas. You had to guess by the sailing time and how stiff your socks were.'

'Sounds horrendous.'

'It was alright. A great gang of fellers. Although I was taller than the others so my feet stuck out the cot.'

He winds his shirt sleeve back down, neatly buttons it at the wrist.

'You was properly on your own, though,' he says. 'Which sounds funny, given how crowded we were. It all took a bit of adjustment.'

'I'm not sure I'd have lasted.'

'You got weeded out beforehand. Put through your paces. Although sometimes it got too much and someone flipped. I remember one guy, we had to pull him off the hatch he was swinging off it, shouting and screaming. We had to knock him out with happy pills and drop him off a week later to a passing ship. Never did see him again. No one blamed him. It could get to you, that's for sure. It weren't like topside. It weren't like the skimmers.'

'How d'you mean?'

'Well – y'see? – it was all so top secret. They used to adapt the submarine before we went out. In case we got caught. They used to paint out all the numbers, on the tower and whatnot. And they used to take off anything that weren't strictly necessary, to save weight. They even stripped out the rescue buoys – y'know? – the things you'd launch to mark your position if you got stuck down there. If you did – God help you – no other fucker would. There wouldn't be anyone launching no rescue missions. That was it. The powers that be would shrug and deny all knowledge. Like it never happened. Like you never existed.'

He stares at me.

'And now look! I fall over in the bathroom and five minutes later the bloody cavalry are riding through the door.'

Joan is lying in bed, a beanie wrap-around cushion supporting her neck, her long white hair wild on her shoulders.

'I'm quite alright as I am, thank you,' she says fussing ineffectually at the sheets. 'I don't want anything.'

Joan is ninety-five, tiny, translucent, tethered to the world by her watch and her will and the pictures on the wall.

'I had a twin brother,' she says, not to me, I don't think, particularly, or anyone else in the room I can see. 'Flew with the RAF.

Never came back.'

'Sorry to hear that.'

She doesn't react.

I've come to see how Joan is after her fall yesterday. The ambulance picked her up, although a mouse could've done it. I can't imagine Joan falling – or at least, only as a dried leaf might fall, slowly, with a soundless settling to the forest floor.

'I was an hour older,' she says, closing her eyes, to bring it clearer to mind. Then adds: 'It's a little more than that now.'

❧

Jack is sitting at the kitchen table, the bright morning sunshine intensifying the yellows and greens of his tracksuit, and the silvery lustre of his magnificent, Edwardian, handlebar moustache.

'You don't look ninety-five,' I tell him. 'If you'd have said seventy-five, maybe.'

'Who do I make the cheque out to?' he asks, then takes a sip of tea. 'No – really – that's most awfully kind of you to say so,' he adds, carefully sweeping his moustache for drips, once to the left and once to the right.

There's a helium balloon tied to the corner of his chair.

'Happy Birthday for the other day!' I tell him.

'Thank you,' says Jack, closing his eyes and nodding. 'D'you know – the funny thing is – I never really celebrated birthdays. They used to pass me by, quite unnoticed.'

'That's a shame.'

'It just never seemed that important to me. Perhaps that's why I've reached this preposterous age. I lost track of how old I was sometime around thirty.'

'Well – whatever the reason, I'm very impressed. I hope I'm as good when I get to ninety-five. If I ever do.'

'Oh – you'll be fine,' he says, finishing off the tea and wiping his moustache again. 'Of course, there are no guarantees.'

'Did you score any good presents?'

'Do you know I can't remember!' he says, then folds his arms and leans back. 'I tell you one birthday present I do remember, though. The best one I ever had. No doubt you'll think me quite daft.'

'What was it?'

'It was nineteen forty-one. I was eighteen or thereabouts. On a warship somewhere in the Atlantic. Well – one of the chaps got wind of the fact it was my birthday. Why didn't you tell us he said. We'd have made a fuss. And he hurried off. The next thing I knew, he'd come back with an enormous tin of plums. Greengages, in syrup. He'd been to the kitchen, you see, and made a fuss about it being my birthday and so on, and that's what they had spare. So we took the plums up on deck, to the sunniest spot we could find. And we sat down and we ate them with our fingers, one after the other. It doesn't sound like much, but it meant the world to me.'

'I like plums.'

'Yes, well, there were rather a lot,' he says. 'You'd have been alright.'

'That reminds me of a story about my Uncle John,' I tell him. 'He'd been fighting in Italy when he got captured and thrown in a POW camp.'

'That's a shame,' says Jack. 'Was he a marine?'

'No. Regular army. Anyway, the story goes he escaped from the camp and fought with the partisans.'

'Good man!'

'Yeah – but the thing is, when I asked Auntie Ollie about it, she said that wasn't what happened at all. She said he shacked up with a farmer's daughter and finished the war picking peaches. It's a shame I don't get the chance to see her more often. She's all the way down in Exmouth.'

Jack looks startled.

'I heard the exact same story!'

'Did you?'

'Yes! My wife came from Devon. One of those villages where you can't walk five paces without bumping into a second cousin or what have you. Now, Rachel's brother – one of her brothers – he disappeared in the war and they all thought the worst. But then he turned up in the Woolpack with nothing more than a grin and a pocket full of peach pits.'

Jack strokes his moustache, then slaps the table.

'I'll bet you a pound to a pinch of snuff it was the same farm!' he says.

✑

'Goodness!' says Ian, opening the door. 'There must be a line of you waiting out in the street!'

'It's like that, sometimes. Especially at the beginning. We all tend to just pile in.'

'And a jolly good thing it is, too!' he says, showing me inside. 'I must say, it's been rather overwhelming. But in a good way – you know. In a good way.'

He shows me through to his mother, Peggy, who is propped up on several pillows, doing The Times crossword. She sets the newspaper aside to shake my hand, takes off her reading glasses and puts them on the bedside table next to a porcelain saucer with one partially nibbled, white chocolate biscuit.

'So kind of you to come,' she says. 'Do please have a seat. Is there anything we can get you?'

I tell her I'm fine. She smiles and then nods at Ian, who almost seems to give a little bow before turning and quietly leaving the room.

'I'll just be out here,' he says.

'Thank you, darling,' says Peggy. Then once he's gone, she adds: 'I'd be lost without him.'

Peggy is almost a hundred years old. Although she's been pretty independent up until a month ago, it's all suddenly caught up with her, and now her body is starting to fail in earnest, the flesh retreating from her bones in the most cruelly anatomical way, revealing all the hollows and protuberances, the cords of her neck, the scoop of her temples. Her eyes are still bright, though, as I've no doubt they always were – she seems such a poised and intelligent woman – but perhaps with a cooler, more intense grade of light, the fire of a star at night.

'I was just admiring your frogs,' I tell her after introducing myself and unpacking my things.

'Yes. Aren't they a wonder?' she says. 'I used to spend hours out there, crouched down by the edge, watching them come and go. I'm sure the neighbours thought I was quite potty. But there's no shortage of things to admire in nature, don't you find?'

'I certainly do. We've got a wildlife pond at home.'

'Have you?'

'Lots of frogs. Newts, too.'

'And all those marvellous insects, skimming about on the surface...'

'You're right! No shortage of things to look at.'

'Yes!'

'Do they make much noise, your frogs?'

'No, not really. Except in mating season, when they all get terribly exercised. Or when one of the cats fetches one out, which is horrible, of course, and I've tried my damndest to stop them. We haven't got any newts, though, so I'm jealous on that score. I do so love my frogs!'

I conduct the examination, and everything is pretty much as expected, given the circumstances.

'Well, one thing's for sure,' says Peggy, suddenly serious. 'I will not be going to hospital. You can do whatever else you like with me, but I will not be agreeing to that.'

'No. I understand.'

'I mean – for goodness sake! Look at me! Whatever is the point?'

'You are the boss of you, Peggy. We'll do whatever's best for you.'

'That's kind,' she says. 'It's so easy to get swept up in these things sometimes – don't you find?'

'Absolutely.'

As I'm filling out the paperwork, I ask her what she did when she was working.

'I messed about in the government during the war. Started off in the typing pool but after one thing and another found myself in the Foreign Office, helping out in the Middle East. All frightfully interesting. I travelled about quite a bit afterwards, of course. There was nothing I liked better when I had a bit of free time than to stick out my thumb and hitchhike. I travelled right the way through Syria like that. Fascinating country. Breaks my heart to see what's happening there now, of course. Those poor people.'

'Did you hitchhike on your own?'

'Of course!' she says, 'although, these days...' and she spreads her arms wide and smiles just as broadly, 'I don't suppose I'd get all that far!'

'I've never been what you might call quiet,' says Elsa, tugging the bedclothes up around her neck. 'That's one thing you could never accuse me of. I suppose you're either a talker or you're not. You never have to worry about awkward silences with me. It's just the way I'm built. Like being left-handed. Or having a head for heights.'

I'm waiting with Elsa for the ambulance to come. I'd been sent round for an initial assessment, ECG and bloods. But it was clear as soon as I walked in the bedroom that Elsa was acutely unwell. A closer examination led me to suspect she was suffering a serious internal bleed, so I called 999.

'They'll be here soon,' I told her, putting the phone down. Try not to worry. Meanwhile, I'll get a few things together.'

It's been a while, now. Three-quarters of an hour.

When I go next door to phone ambulance control for an update, I'm told that they're doing their best, an ambulance will be dispatched just as soon as one is available – only, people are having heart attacks, strokes…. surely I can understand? I know it's difficult, I tell him, but the fact remains, we need to get Elsa to hospital as soon as possible.

She's compensating reasonably well at the moment, but I don't think that'll last much longer. We're doing our best, they say. Of course, I say. I appreciate your help.

When I hang up I carefully document the delay.

'Not long now,' I tell Elsa, going back into the bedroom.

Before what, I wonder. She looks so fragile, lying on the bed like this, the sockets of her eyes ghosting through the pallid stretch of her face.

'I'm glad you're here,' she says. 'I wouldn't want to do this on my own.'

'I'm glad I'm here, too,' I tell her, sitting beside her to do another set of obs. 'So – go on. You were telling me about Stars in Battledress…'

'I was always mad about the stage,' she says. 'Singing, dancing, doing sketches. And that was what they wanted. A friend of mine put me up to it. She said I was just the kind of girl they were looking for. It was such a shame what happened to her.'

'Why? What happened?'

'It was a famous murder case. She was on a cruise ship coming back from a show in South Africa and she was murdered by one of the ship stewards. He tried to make out she'd agreed to have sex with him, but then died of a fit or something, and he panicked and shoved her body out of the porthole. They never did find her body. He was convicted, of course. I think he only escaped hanging because of some loophole or other. Died in prison, years later. Funny how these things work out. Poor Gay. She was such a kind girl, a lovely girl. But these things happen, I suppose. On a ship or anywhere else. You've just got to be careful and lucky and hope for the best.'

Elsa tells me about the shows she was in. One in particular.

'As well as performing, everyone had a job to do. Mine was to put together these wooden steps for the big dance number in the second half. I was just tightening up the screws when someone dropped a curtain pole straight on my head. Knocked me clean out! When I came to there was only a minute to go before I was on. I had no idea who I was or where I was, but the lights came up, they pointed me in the right direction, and I walked out into the light. Anyway, the words seemed to come from somewhere, so it worked out in the end.'

'When that show was over, I moved into the intelligence corps. I remember – we were all lined up in the corridor, six girls in front, about thirty men behind. You can imagine what that was like. I was the last girl to be called forward. When I heard my name, I thought – right! I'll show these men a thing or two! – so I marched as smartly as I could up to the desk, swinging my arms and hips. But you see, what I didn't realise was there was this rug just in front of the desk, and the floor was highly polished. As soon as my feet touched the rug it flew out from under me and I slid the rest of the way on my arris, disappearing up to my shoulders in the footwell. The Major he stood up and peered over the edge of the desk.

'Are you alright down there?' he said.

'Yes Sir!' I said, and saluted, flat on my back, and everyone laughed. But it didn't do me any harm, apart from a few bruises. They took me on.

The flat door buzzes. I'm relieved to hear it's the ambulance.

Two paramedics walk in.

'Alright?' says one I vaguely recognise. 'Wait a minute… didn't you use to work for us?'

There's a black and white photo of Glenda on the wall taken when she was a young woman in the Land Army. She'd obviously dressed up for the picture, because although she's still in fatigues, her hair is nicely swept back in a wide band, and her lipstick is in a perfect bow. It's a great shot. Glenda's smile is so bright and enthusiastic and full of energy, I can imagine her pulling the spade out of the soil and advancing on the world, waving it overhead.

'They shipped us off to Berkshire,' she says. 'I hated that farmer. We all did. Picking potatoes in the rain. He always used to drive the tractor too quick for us. We couldn't keep up. I used to throw potatoes at him to slow him down. And he'd shout back You throw another one of them fuckin' potatoes at me, Glenda, and you see what happens.'

'And did you?'

'Course I did. He didn't scare me.'

'What happened?'

'We all went on strike. We sat down in the middle of the field and refused to budge. He ranted and raved. You get back to work now or you'll see what for he said. But he was like that. Full of wind.'

'He sounds horrible.'

'Oh – he wasn't too bad once you got to know his ways. He just needed someone to show him who was the real boss round there. I remember this one time, I was up on a hay rick and I saw a mouse. Well – if there's one thing I absolutely detest and cannot abide, it's a mouse. But where you goin' to run when you're standing on the top of a hay rick? You silly cow – it's only a fucking mouse he said. You come up here and deal with it, if you're such an expert I said, and threw the pitchfork at him. But he didn't know, you see? He didn't know how much I hate mice. And rats. I can't stand rats.'

'Maybe he should've got a dog. To catch the rats.'

'He did have a dog, a Jack Russell, called Gravel. Vicious, pointy little thing.'

'So I'm guessing you didn't have such a great time in the Land Army then?'

'Oh no. We had a great laugh. There was a prisoner of war camp down the road, full of Eye-talians. We used to hang around the fence and pass carrots through the wire. 'Ere. Get away from there! the guards used to say. Drop them carrots! Didn't bother us, though. They needed fresh food and attention. And so did we.'

Whilst we're talking, there's a sudden, soggy thump behind me, like an albatross just flew into the window.

'Window man's here,' says Glenda, easing her position in the chair. 'They have to do it on a long pole these days, ever since the last one fell off his ladder. D'you know something? I was brought up in a tenement block in Ladbroke Grove. Six floors up we were. And every Sunday my mum used to sit out on the ledge to clean the outside. Hold me legs, Glenda she used to say. And I'd be hanging on for dear life, her stockings slipping down, and I'd be shouting For God's sake, Mum. Haven't you finished yet? I'm losing yah! And she'd shout back Don't be so silly, Glenda. Just hold me legs! Her voice all muffled like, because she was the other side of the window, and I had one ear in her lap. And she'd be out there, cheerful as you like, scrubbing the window singing away as easy as if she was polishing the mirror in the bathroom. She was good, my mum. And she certainly had a head for heights.'

Glenda seems distracted for a moment, brushing some biscuit crumbs from her lap.

'And you might not think to look at me now,' she carries on at last. 'But I tell you what – I had one hell of a grip.'

'Anchored off Syracuse. Everyone fucker below deck drowned. Boom. Gone. That was a hard business. 'Course – I was sleeping on top, so at least I had a chance. At least I could make a swim for it.'

Frankie's eyes are so hooded, and the way the light is in the room, it's almost as if he doesn't have eyes at all. That, and his habit of moving his bottom jaw from side to side when he's not talking, makes him seem like a statue chewing over the hard facts of his life.

'Them kind of things mattered, where you slept and everything. I've always been a good sleeper. I could sleep upside down on a washing line. I used to sleep under the truck, so long as the ground was hard enough. Gave you a measure of protection. Here, they said. Frankie. Take these trucks up the coast for us. We drove from Port Said to Damascus. Had a whale of a time. We used to mix it up, course. Well – we was young, mate. We had nothing to lose. We knew we was basically cattled.'

He narrows his dark eyes at me and grinds his teeth.

'D'you know what I mean? Cattled? That's cockney slang, mate.

Cattle trucked. Fucked.'

He laughs, settles back in the chair.

'My missus was the brains of the operation. She was in the Waaf. There weren't nothing she couldn't do. Ride a motorbike. Shoot down a plane. Unscramble a secret message. I tell you what, I landed on my feet all right the day I met Junie.'

He grinds his teeth again and shifts his position in the chair.

'She's in a home now. I don't see her all that much. Even when I do she don't recognise me. That's the dementia for you, mate. Still – I keep her bed made up. That way I reckon there's a chance she might come back.'

Kenneth's house is so ancient and well-heeled it has its name stencilled on the curving corner brickwork of the street. Black railings lead round from the sign beneath tall windows to the porticoed entrance, three wide steps up to a black and white tiled threshold, a wide oak door and worn brass bell-pull. The keysafe to the side is a glaring modern expediency whose installation I imagine took some persuading, but given Kenneth's age and poor state of health I'm glad he agreed. When I'd called earlier to arrange a time, Kenneth told me to retrieve the key and let myself in. 'I'll be in the drawing room,' he said, room pronounced rum. 'Just holler out when you're in the hall so I'll know it's you,' he said. 'There's a fellow.'

The hall is as sumptuous as you'd expect from the exterior. A wide, softly curving staircase, smooth as the whorled interior of a whelk, rising on plush red treads past paintings, prints by Gillray, fading family pictures dating from the age of the plate, up past a gilt and crystal chandelier to the honey-moted tones of the upper storeys. Another jarring note, though – the stair lift, whose track starts by a walnut table for keys and things, where there's a silver framed photograph of Kenneth as a young airman, leaning forward in that earnest, David Niven way, cap jauntily back, arms crossed and resting

67

on an immaculately pressed trouser leg.

'Up here!' he says when I call – then subsides into a series of rattling coughs.

I squeeze past the chair where it's come to a stop at the top of the stairs, and walk into a bright and beautiful room, where Kenneth is waiting for me in his favourite chair.

'Thank you so much for coming,' he says, shaking my hand. 'Do take a pew.'

Kenneth's observations are below normal range but it's unsurprising, given his COPD and recent chest infection.

'It doesn't help that I smoked for fifty years or more,' he wheezes. 'Well everybody did. It was almost compulsory. And during the war one tended to live day to day. I loved to smoke, though. It was one of the few things I was good at. If I didn't have a cigarette, I'd smoke a pipe. And if I didn't have any pipe tobacco, I'd jolly well cut up some old carpet and smoke that. I managed to quit in the end, though.'

'How did you manage it?'

'Funny story. My wife had arranged a family trip. A pauper's experience of Paris she called it. Didn't sound at all like my cup of tea but I went along with it as I often did. I'd read George Orwell of course. Down and Out in Paris and London. Marvellous book. I remember him talking about the twopenny hangover, which was a rope you could lean on whilst you were sitting on a bench. And then at the end of the night they'd untie the rope, and there you were! Orwell smoked like the proverbial, of course. Didn't do him any good either, although I think he had a touch of the old TB. Anyway, there we were, checking into this blackened ruin in the Place de la Contrescarpe – or the Can't Escape, as I called it. Awful. Indescribable. And I remember lying there that night, staring up at the ceiling, smoking cigarette after cigarette – A because I couldn't think what else to do and B because I thought it might discourage the fleas. And I thought to myself Kenneth! What on earth are you doing, lying here like this, killing yourself! So we checked out and went somewhere a little more civilised. I gave my last pack of Chesterfields to the person sleeping in the doorway, and I never smoked again. And now here you are telling me my breathing's no good!'

'Well – it's not great.'

'I'm ninety-five, Jim. I don't think you could truthfully describe any aspect of me as being great. But there we are. You're a smashing fellow and I thank you for your time.'

4: *Alternate Realities*

'Peter died six years ago, but it may as well be six minutes.'

'I'm so sorry for your loss.'

She shrugs.

'Oh, well. I had a long time to get used to the idea. Poor Peter. He was a long time sick, you see. But that's all in the past. D'you know what I miss the most? The conversations we had. About the silliest things, any time of the day or night. He was a fascinating man, Peter. That's why I married him, I think. Or one of the reasons. He would always go to great lengths to understand the other person's point of view. His hospital bed was just there, where you are now, and I was off to the side, reading or dozing or running backwards and forwards to let the carers in, the nurses and so on. The number of people who came and went through this room. I could've written a book. Should've. And now it's just me, sitting on my own, staring out at the birds, thinking about not very much.'

'Do you have family?'

'No. Not really. All my brothers and sisters are gone now and we didn't want children. There are some nieces and nephews dotted about. I see them from time to time, which is lovely, but they've got busy lives and what have you and I don't want to burden them. I don't mind. I'm perfectly content. No – we didn't really want children, and I never gave it any thought. I did have a strange dream about it, though. I'd fallen asleep in this chair, and I woke up inside the dream, so to speak. I could tell, because even though everything was much the same, the light was different, more – I don't know – electric. And there was a wild infant child standing to the side of me. A girl. She was standing right there, just about where you are now, rocking from side to side and staring at me. I wasn't frightened or anything. I just held out my hand, and eventually she came forward, and let me stroke her hair a while. Then something startled her, and she ran out through the open window into the garden, which was so thick with trees it was like a tropical jungle. And she ran off into all that, and I watched her go. But I wasn't worried for her, because I knew she would be safe out there, among all the animals, the bears and the wolves and so on. You read about those children, don't you? The feral ones, the ones who run off into the forest and get brought up by animals.'

'I remember something about that. It's difficult to know whether it's a story or just neglect. Probably a bit of both.'

'Yes. There is that. People often make up stories when the truth is too painful.'

Jack's directions to the block are a strange mixture of precise and vague.

'We're the one with the flapping green canopy,' he says. 'The last brick building on the right as you head up from the sea. No – wait a minute. What am I saying? Second to last. But hang on – there are lots of brick buildings between us and the top road. But anyway. Flapping green canopy. Look for that.'

He's right about the canopy. I can only think that all the recent bad weather has partially torn it from its fixings. I locate Jack and Morag's flat among the forty or so others, press the buzzer, and wait – for so long I wonder if it's working. Just before I press it again a voice crackles on the speaker.

'Hello, Jack,' I say, leaning in, struggling to be heard over the wind and the canopy. 'It's Jim. From the hospital.'

'Right you are, Jim. Come on up.'

He buzzes the door and I push through.

Just as I turn to close it, I see a woman walking up the path. She's zippered to the chin in a metallic blue anorak with just her face showing from the hood of it, carrying a cat-patterned shopping bag in one hand and a Cornish pasty in the other. I hold the door for her and wait. She doesn't acknowledge me at all, just walks and eats, walks and eats, dividing her attention between the pasty and the pavement. She's so methodical about the whole thing she reminds me of a cartoon robot, analysing a sample of human food whilst she makes her way back to the mothership.

'There you go!' I say, as she plods through the door. 'I can see you've got your hands full.'

She walks past me without making the slightest acknowledgement – so ruthlessly I imagine she would have simply smashed through the door if I hadn't been standing there to open it – scattering pastry crumbs as she heads for the lift, which happens to be ready waiting. By the time I've picked all my bags up, both robot pasty woman and lift have gone.

I walk up.

Jack looks exactly as he sounds: pressed trousers, green cardigan, small check shirt and tie, silvery hair flowing backwards like the ripples in a crinkle cut chip.

'Found us alright?' he says, silently closing the door. 'Morag's in the sitting room. Last door on the left. Sorry – my left. As you look at the window.'

You would absolutely match them if they were playing cards. Morag is a watchful, bird-like woman, perfectly turned out in a silk blouse and tartan skirt, with crinkly hair that goes side to side rather than straight back.

'Who is it, Jack...?' she says, gripping the arms of the armchair.

'Just a nurse from the hospital, darling,' he says. 'No need to be alarmed.'

She turns her clear blue eyes on me and waits to see what I'll do.

'So – how are you feeling, Morag?'

'How am I feeling?'

'Yes. In yourself.'

She frowns at me, as if that's the most extraordinary thing anyone's ever asked her.

'I know you've had quite a day of it,' I say.

'Have I?'

'Well – coming home from the hospital. After a long stay. Must be nice to be home.'

She shakes her head, sharing her bewilderment between me and Jack.

'It's alright, darling,' he says. 'Nothing to worry about. You're home now.'

'I am, aren't I?'

'Yes. And it's lovely to have you back.'

Jack smiles at me with a level of control as perfect as his hair.

'I've been sent by the hospital just to make sure you have everything you need, Morag,' I say. 'And to see what we can to do help. By way of equipment, physiotherapy, nursing – anything really. We want to make sure you're safe, that's all.'

'I have everything, thank you,' she says, with great precision.

Whilst the laptop warms up, and to keep the conversation going, I ask Morag if there's anything troubling her.

'There is, actually.'

'Oh yes? What's that?'

'I've been having bad dreams.'

'I'm sorry to hear that, Morag. What kind of bad dreams?'

'There are these people. Young people. And they keep wandering in and out. Sometimes they look at me. Sometimes they don't. Sometimes they walk straight past, carrying things. Pushing things. And I haven't the faintest idea who they are or what they want.'

'That was the hospital, darling,' says Jack, patting her on the hand. 'That was the hospital.'

Stella has known Glad for quite a few years. More than she cares to think about. Lately their friendship's been under something of a strain, though. Glad has become increasingly obsessed with her dolls – expensive, hyper-realistic babies with internal motors that give them a heartbeat and make them breathe. The dolls are so authentically painted and well-made, you'd never know they were fake until you got up close.

'Her son gets them for her – why, I couldn't possibly say,' says Stella. 'They cost an absolute packet. You have to send away for them. To America or somewhere. She spends hours going over the details, telling them what she wants. Then he buys them with his credit card. I don't know what he thinks about it all. He's an only child. It must mean something.'

It's interesting, talking to Stella about this. We're sitting in her front room, a warm, slightly down-at-heel place with overstuffed sofas, bookshelves, a coffee table with TV magazines and remote controls, a dog curled up in a fleecy bed. Unlike Glad, Stella's had lots of children. Their photographs line the walls, glimpses of the usual family situations: holidays, weddings, graduations, babies. It's all so real. I can imagine sending away for it, and then waiting for the delivery, everything flat-packed, ready to assemble, even the dog (batteries not included).

'It makes me so uncomfortable,' Stella goes on. 'She puts them in a pram and takes them for a walk round the park, even the play area. People come over to have a look because of course they think she's just a grandma helping out with the kids. And then when they see that they're dolls, well, they pull away. I think they think she's got dementia. Maybe she has. The other day one of the parents called the police. They turned up at her house to talk to her about it. They didn't do anything, though – well, Glad says they took it in turns to hold the baby and take photos, but that was it. I don't know. It's all a bit weird.'

I'm looking through Judy's notes, the last time someone listened to her chest. I can't help laughing.

'What's so funny?' she says.

'Well – I think the nurse who wrote this must've been hungry. She's written bilateral crepes.'

I show her the little drawing in the notes. The rough sketch of her lungs, a line of little crosses at the bottom of both, an arrow pointing to them.

Judy's expression doesn't change.

'What does that mean?' she says.

'It should say creps.'

'Craps?'

'Creps. Short for crepitations. I think that's what it stands for. Anyway, it's that crackly sound you get sometimes when there's gunk in the lungs.'

Judy shrugs.

'I know all about that,' she says. 'I've had enough of that.'

'You're sounding better today, though.'

'I'm not dead yet, then?'

'No! Alive and kicking.'

'I'll kick you in a minute.'

'I wouldn't mind.'

She stares at me.

'Where are you from?' she says. 'Or-stralia?'

'Australia? No! I was born in London but brought up in the Fens.'

'Oh,' she says. 'That explains it.'

I shut the folder and carry on with the examination.

Judy is ninety-eight but looks older. In fact, with her quilted housecoat, netted, silvery hair, enormous slippers, stiffly jointed movements – the way she wobbles along clinging to a kitchen trolley loaded with toast, Tommy Tippee beaker and emergency button – it feels like I'm in a marionette update of the Red Riding Hood story, where the Big Bad Wolf works for a Community Health Team, and lets himself in with a silver key from the keysafe.

'Are you going to be much longer?' she says.

'No. Almost done.'

She takes a toot of tea from the beaker.

'Would you like me to freshen that up for you?'

'No – thank you,' she says. 'I shall need the lavatory.'

There's a pause whilst I add my notes to the folder.

'What did you do – before you retired?' I say.

'Shorthand typist,' she says.

'How lovely!' I say. 'I like typing. It's one of the most useful skills I ever learned. That and driving.'

'I worked in a brewery,' she says, moving on. 'That's where I met Alf.'

'Did he work in the office, too?'

'Nah. He was in and out. But we'd throw things at each other and we sort of went on from there.'

'Sounds brilliant.'

'It was hard during the war, though. Terrible hard. There were these Ack Ack guns on the roof. You should've heard 'em when they went off. Boom! Boom! Boom! The whole place shook like it was gonna fall in. They were having a pop at all them German bombers comin' over. It was a terrible business. Terrible.'

'How long were you married, Judy?'

'A long time. So long I couldn't tell ya. But Alf's been gone for years now and – well – that's that.'

'I'm sorry.'

'What for? It's not your fault. Is it?'

'No. I suppose not.'

'Well then.'

I put the finishing touches to the notes.

'Why don't you go upstairs and have a lie-down if you're tired?' she says.

I look up from the folder.

'Sorry, Judy – what?'

'Not you,' she says. 'Him.'

She narrows her eyes and nods at the empty chair behind me. I turn to look.

'My old man,' she says, sighing and leaning back again. 'If I don't keep talking to him, he might go orf' with someone else.'

❦

Minnie opens the door.

'Good morning,' she says. 'Please. Come in.'

As soon as I'm in the hall I slip my shoes off.

'My word! You are domesticated!' she says, then formally gestures to one of her kitchen chairs. 'Do take a seat.

Despite the painful crook of her back, the palsied tremor of her head and the general wear and tear of her ninety-eight years, Minnie is remarkably chipper.

'I was a dancer,' she says as I go through the examination. 'Ballet first, then contemporary. Although you wouldn't think it to look at me now.'

I don't agree, though. There's a poise to her that suggests years of training and performance. It certainly goes some way to explaining her sparkling demeanour. I imagine she'd jump up if I asked her and attempt a pirouette on the spot, sweeping all her medications off the table with a velcro slipper.

'And when my performance days were done, I went into dance therapy. D'you know, when I used to say that to people, they'd often say Ah yes! That's when you put your arms out and tell them to be a tree. Be a tree, they'd say! But of course, they'd got it completely wrong. The only thing that can be a tree is a tree! No – what you say is: Think about a tree. Now – hold that feeling, and let it start to move you. D'you see the difference?'

I tell her I do, that it's a subtle distinction but a good one.

'Or they'd say Be a boat on a wavy sea! What utter nonsense! They don't know what they're talking about.'

We go through the examination. Apart from some recent dizziness, everything seems pretty good.

'Yes, well, the family was blessed with old bones. Or cursed, I'm not sure,' she says, buttoning up her sleeve. 'My two elder sisters are both gone now, poor souls, but they lived to their hundreds. I don't doubt Agatha could've gone on a lot longer, but she fell out with her doctor, threw away her pills and that was that.'

At the end of it all I shake her warmly by the hand.

'Lovely to meet you, Minnie,' I say.

'You too, dear,' she says. 'Now don't forget your shoes.'

Back at the hospital, I'm in the middle of handing over my patients for the day.

'Ah, now – Minnie!' I say, pulling out her report. 'She was an absolute delight!'

Jess, one of the nurses, is sitting right behind me. She turns round in her chair and leans forward to look over my shoulder.

'Thought so,' she says. 'There aren't too many Minnies around. Thank God.'

'Why? What d'you mean? Didn't you like her?'

'No. She was absolutely vile. Her and her daughter.'

'What happened?'

'I phoned her up to arrange an appointment. Two o'clock alright? I said. Fine, lovely. Great. See you then, sort of thing. So I get there dot on two and knock and knock and ring the bell. Nothing, no reply. I phone the landline. No answer. And I'm looking around, wondering what to do, just about to call the office to get some advice when I hear a rumble from inside, and when I look through the letterbox I can see someone coming down on the chair lift. Well – eventually after about ten years the door flies open. What the hell d'you think you're playing at! she says. I was upstairs having my nap. So I say how sorry I am to have disturbed her and everything, but I did phone and ask what time. She completely ignores that, of course. You people just think you can barge in any time of the day or night. Rah rah rah. To be honest I'm so shocked by all of this I just stand there and take it – and that's when her daughter comes running over from the Co-op. Have you met Minnie's daughter?'

'No. I saw a picture of her on the wall though. She looks nice.'

'Nice? Satan in a bad wig and red lippy kinda nice. She comes racing over, stopping the traffic, apples everywhere. What d'you think you're doing? she's shouting. Who are you? Why wasn't I informed? and so on. And everyone in the street's stopping to look, like I'm some kind of evil bailiff or something, come to turf them out of their house.'

'Oh. Well. I'm shocked.'

'So go on, then. How come she was nice to you and so horrible to me?'

'I don't know,' I said. 'Maybe she's worse when the daughter's there?'

'Hmm,' says Jess, turning back to her desk. 'Maybe. Or maybe it's just a two o'clock monster kinda deal.'

I'd been worried about taking this assessment so late in the day. There are often snags, so many things that can go wrong, and you can find yourself struggling to make it all right long after your finishing time. But as I hurry back to the car with all my things, checking my watch, rehearsing the best route to the hospital to beat the evening traffic, I can't help thinking it had all gone so much better than I could have hoped. In fact, it had been an ideal kind of assessment. Maud had been a charming patient, radiantly pleased to be home again after a couple of weeks in hospital, stroking the arms of her favourite chair like she fully expected them to close around her in a welcoming hug. The Red Cross ambulance crew that brought her home had been as meticulously kind and attentive as you could possibly get without actually hiring them from a catalogue called Angels in the Community. They'd even bought a week's shopping for her, ready meals, bread, margarine and long-life milk, and put it all neatly away. There had been no medical complications. There was mention in the hospital referral of neighbours who were active in her support. So all in all, it had taken very little sorting out, and I had a reasonable chance of finishing on time.

I'm sitting in the car with the window down, putting my sunglasses on and turning the engine over ready to set off, when a door across the road opens and an anguished woman hurries out. Her hair is dyed a dusky yellow and held in a clump straight up by a thick green band, making her look like an anguished pineapple. She is barefoot.

'Have you seen Maud?' she pants.

'Yes. I've just finished there. I'm from the hospital.'

'Good. Then I need to talk to you,' she says – and then waits for me to turn the engine off again and get out of the car, glancing up and down the street, one hand on the roof, like she's ready to hold me back if I decide to make a dash for it.

'What's the problem?' I say when I'm out, leaning back against the car.

'A terrible thing happened,' she says.

'What terrible thing? When?'

'We've known her for years. We all of us have. We're in and out all the time. Well it's like that round here. It's a very friendly street. We look out for each other. I must have twenty keys in my kitchen. Can you feed the cat? Can you water the plants?'

'So – what's this terrible thing?'

'We couldn't do enough for her. There's me, there's my husband Nikolai. There's Enda. She's a retired nurse. Her nerves are shot. We've picked Maud off the floor. We've gone to the supermarket twice a week. Got the paper, fixed her water when she had that flood. We've moved furniture. We've done just about everything for that woman...'

'Sorry – I don't even know your name...'

'Gloria. I'm Gloria,' she says, holding out her hand. I shake it. It feels soft and damp.

'Do you think we should talk about this inside, Gloria?'

'Yes, of course.'

She pads back across the road with the high, tentative steps and arms out to the side like a holidaymaker on the beach. Her husband Nikolai – I'm guessing it's him – has appeared at the door. He's the exact opposite of Gloria – monosyllabic, graven. He squeezes my hand in his great, fleshy paw of a hand, whilst dropping his other hand weightily onto my shoulder at the same time, making me buckle on that side.

'Come!' he says. 'Would you like drink? Eat?'

'That's kind,' I say, starting to feel desperate. 'But I can't be long.'

'Nonsense!' says Nikolai. 'I get you something.'

He thumps off into the back kitchen whilst Gloria carries on with her frantic monologue in the lounge.

''... because of course we none of us mind doing any of these things for Maud. I've had elderly parents. Nikolai's father. The Tremletts next door, the Parkinsons at number eight. We've been there for them. Because that's what we'd expect for ourselves, and we'd do it all again in a heartbeat. But then this thing happened and I can't tell you... it's horrible.... awful....'

'What happened? I have to be quick, only...'

'All these years. Thirty-eight years. And the irony is, we've paid out quite a bit. We ran a kind of tab, you know? A week's shopping, bits and pieces for the house. She'd get one bill or another and of course she doesn't have any cards or a bank account so it'd be Gloria – do you think you could sort this out for me and we'll settle up at the end of the month. And sometimes she would, and sometimes she wouldn't.'

'Has she accused you of stealing money?'

Gloria blanches and stops talking, and for a second I think she's going to faint.

'It was awful,' she says. 'Terrible. Horrible. You see, she's so paranoid about burglars. She's getting worse. Isn't she, Nikolai?'

He's coming back into the room with a tray of tea and a plate of tiny square pastries.

'Here. Come,' he says, putting the tray on the coffee table and then gesturing to the sofa. I sink down onto it, take a pastry. And maybe it's because I'm hot and a little wired, but this pastry is far and away the driest, sweetest thing I've ever put in my mouth, a triple honey, sugared pistachio desiccant sachet.

'Mmm,' I say, half-choking and hurriedly reaching for my tea. 'Thanks. So – then what happened?'

'We went to see her in hospital. Didn't we, Nikolai?'

'Ye-es!' he says, spreading his hands. 'Of course!'

'So she was saying all this and that about her house. How many people knew she was away. Who had a key and who didn't. So I said to her: Come on, Maud. We've all been friends for donkeys' years. And she said Yes, but I don't know – you might have relatives who are burglars.'

Nikolai pops a pastry in his mouth like it's really nothing at all, and smacks his hands.

'Aah!' he says, then wipes his beard.

'No, Nikolai,' says Gloria, like she understands the real meaning behind that gesture. 'I know she's ninety-five, but there's nothing wrong with her up here,' she says, tapping the side of her head. 'Nothing at all. And that's what makes it so hard to take. I mean it'd be alright if she had dementia. If you know what I mean.'

'I know what you mean,' I say, red in the face. The tea is superheated, but I have to drink as much of it as I can so as not to appear rude.

'So then she says Oh Gloria – I've got all that money upstairs. And all my rings. Could you take care of it for me? So I said Of course I will, Maud. And the first thing I did when I got back from the hospital, I went over there, and I got it all together in one big envelope – and it had to be a big envelope, because there was eleven hundred pound in total – eleven hundred! – and you can count it yourself if you don't believe me. And I put it all safe here. And the next day when we went back to see her, I told her what I'd done. And honestly, Jim – you should've seen her face. I didn't tell you to take my money! she said, everyone looking, all the nurses and people. What have you done, stealing all my money! I've a good mind to call the police on you. Well! I felt so sick. I wanted the floor to open up and swallow me whole.'

'She was upset,' says Nikolai, closing his eyes and slowly shaking his head.

'I said to her I'm perfectly happy to put it all back for you, Maud. I was only trying to help. So I came straight back, got the envelope and put everything back how it was. And I haven't been in to see her since, because I can't have that hanging over me. I can't expose myself to accusations like that, can I? I mean – what d'you think? You do your best for someone and then this happens.'

I tell her that she's quite right to withdraw contact, at least for the time being, until things settle down. I tell her I'll report back to the nurse in charge, and we'll come up with a plan.

'We'll be putting in temporary care and so on, so you don't have to worry about that. And I'll have a word with the social workers to see what they think.'

Gloria tells me about the effect all this is having on the other neighbour, Enda, and Nikolai starts to pour me another cup of tea – so I have to act decisively if I'm not to be caught here for another hour.

'Thank you so much for the tea and everything – and for being so frank about what happened,' I say, backing towards the door, the two of them standing together and advancing on me. I reach out and shake their hands in an effort to underline the fact that the meeting is over. Nikolai holds on to my hand, though, alternating a squeeze with a nod of his head and a closing of his eyes. I squeeze his hand back, but still he doesn't release, and it goes on for an interminable length of time, until I manage to free my hand and move purposefully to the front door.

'Bye then.'

Gloria follows me outside and across the road, still in her bare feet.

I open the car door by touch and slip inside, winding down the window to make some allowance for the fact that Gloria's still talking.

'That's fine,' I say, starting the engine. 'I know it's easy for me to say, but try not to worry. I think Maud's been upset by her stay in hospital. It can be quite disorienting, and she is pretty elderly. Anyway – it's been lovely to meet you.'

I put on my sunglasses.

'I'm really sorry, though, Gloria – I have to go now.'

'Yes,' she says. 'Of course. You do understand, though, don't you? We've always had her best interests at heart.'

'I can see that,' I tell her. 'I can see you're good neighbours. Try not to worry.'

When I drive away, I catch a glimpse of her in the rear-view mirror, standing forlornly in the middle of the street in her bare feet, looking back at me.

∽

Perched on the edge of her bed, her crochet cap looped over her ears, her smock rucked up, her square face a little wax-yellow in the light from the basement kitchen window, Wendy looks like a character in a painting by Brueghel, the village wise-woman, taking a breather half-way through making the latest batch of crab-apple gin.

'I don't drink the stuff,' she says, wiping her hands down the front of her smock. 'I just like giving it away as presents.'

She gestures to a row of elegant and antique bottles on a shelf behind her. 'There's more in the cellar,' she says. 'Have a look if you like.'

There's nothing I'd like better. I could very happily spend the day exploring this extraordinary house, filled with Wendy's charcoal sketches and stone sculptures and black and white photos and shelf upon shelf of tatty books – the beautiful strata of a long and colourful life lived in many parts of the world. I haven't the time, though. Apart from checking Wendy over and making sure she's okay, I've come to see what we can do to help. We've had a good long chat about the things she could do to improve things environmentally. I've offered to find help with some 'rationalisation' so we can accommodate the hospital bed she desperately needs. Nothing I've said impresses her over much, it has to be said, although she's happy to think about it.

'I like to be in the action,' she says. 'The kitchen is the heart of the house. I don't want to lose that.'

'You wouldn't have to.'

'Hmm,' she says.

She shifts her position, and a batik-print cloth bag rattles out from a pocket onto the cot bed.

'My bones,' she says.

'Your bones? What are you – a necromancer?'

She laughs. 'My phones! My phones! Although – talking about divination – I did see things. In the past. Not so much these days, unfortunately.'

'What kinds of things?'

'Oh – I knew they weren't real. I didn't let myself get frightened by them. And I certainly didn't tell anyone else, or they'd have locked me up! My sister was the same. I think in retrospect it was a form of epilepsy. Only with us it was more hallucinations. When we were little, we both got sent to a convent. Not that anyone had ever told us we were Catholic. What's a Catholic? my sister said to me when we were lined up outside the classroom. I told her to watch out, keep her mouth shut and follow me. Anyway, there was this nun who took us for something or other. She'd slowly write a word on the blackboard, then underline it slowly with two wiggly lines, and finish off by screwing in the chalk to make a dot. And it was that particular sequence, you see, the two wiggly lines, the dot at the end, that would send us off. Animals would burst out of the blackboard. Foxes, eagles, herds of reindeer. We learned to control our surprise or we'd have been for it.'

'Maybe they'd have thought you were visionaries. Is that what they call them?'

'I think if you see the Virgin Mary you're a visionary. Foxes and eagles you're probably a witch. We didn't tell anyone, needless to say.'

'Do you still have visions?'

'Sometimes. Odd times. The last one I was standing at the sink doing some washing up – which dates it! I haven't done that in a while. Anyway, I was standing there with my hands in the sudsy water, and – maybe it was the pattern of light through the window, or something else, I don't know – but suddenly I was standing on the edge of a vast, desert plain. And off in the distance I could see a dummy.'

'A dummy?'

'A tailor's mannequin. On a stand. And I moved closer, and I saw that the dummy was wearing a jacket – a nice, neat, green brocade affair, with pearl buttons down the front and at the cuff. A little closer and I could see some other details, a beetle brooch, a pair of calfskin gloves. And it was then I realised what I was looking at. It's you, you dozy old cow! I said to myself. The vision vanished. I carried on washing up.'

✲

Stephen is telling me about the dream he had last night. He's sitting in his chair looking left towards the windows with his eyes tightly shut, his bony fingers laced in his lap, one long leg crossed over the other, the foot gently bouncing up and down, as if he's judging the weight of the slipper hanging from the toes.

'I've been having these vivid dreams,' he says. 'They're so real it takes me a while to wake up from them. I wondered if it might be the medication.'

'Possibly. What kind of dreams?'

'Last night I was floating in a warm, deep sea. And there were all these people splashing about around me, laughing and shouting. Some I knew, some I didn't. And then I started to sink, down and down and down, not drowning exactly, but not happy about it either. And no-one tried to help me or seemed all that bothered, and everything was getting far away. It was such an odd, lonely feeling. I can't say it was a nightmare, exactly, but I didn't like it all that much. And when I woke up, I found I'd ... had an accident.'

He opens his eyes at that point and twists his mouth into a one-sided smile, cartoon-like, strangely superficial. I can't help thinking he's spent his life practising it.

'The last time I wet the bed must have been seventy years ago, so you can imagine how surprised I was. Still,' he says, his slipper falling to the floor,' I've put something on the mattress tonight, in case I have the sea dream again.'

I pick his slipper up and hang it back on his foot.

'Thank you,' he says. 'Now – what else do you need to know?'

We go over his medical history, medications, recent admission to hospital.

'And of course, no sooner have I come out than Jean goes in. We're like those funny little people on a weather clock.'

'So why has Jean gone to hospital?'

'Didn't they tell you?' he says, closing his eyes and turning his face to the window again. 'I fell on her. She was helping me down the stairs and I lost my balance. Broke her arm in three places. And then they found other things wrong with her, too, in that way they have. So all in all it's been a bit of a disaster.'

Later on, when I've finished all the tests and I'm writing them up, Stephen asks me where I live.

'Oh really?' he says. 'Well it's a shame Jean isn't here, because I think I'm right in saying that's where her grandfather came from. He was a policeman – oh! I'm talking years ago, before the war. I remember her telling me about him. He used to ride around on a motorcycle, like he owned the place. And everyone hated him and his dreadful moustache, which is why they had him killed.'

'Killed? You're kidding? Really?'

'Apparently. Then they all showed up at the funeral, lining the streets with their heads bowed and their hands in front of them, all of them thinking the same thing. Glad to be shot of him.'

'I'll have to look into that.'

'It was a long time ago. The old police station's flats now, apparently. Called Peelers, I think. Funnily enough, that's where I met Jean. At a funeral. She's not my first wife. My first wife died unexpectedly.'

Stephen suddenly opens his eyes and stares straight at me.

'It wasn't her funeral we met at,' he says. 'I don't want you getting the wrong idea.'

'No, no,' I tell him. 'I didn't think it could've been.'

'Good,' he says. 'Because I know how it sounds.'

He finds another cartoon smile, then resumes his blind inspection of the window.

'Yes. Jean looked wonderful in black. She was a hairdresser, down from the North. We got chatting over the cold meat selection, and then shared a cab back to mine. And do you know what I tell people?'

'No? What do you tell them?'

'I tell them it was the only one-night stand I ever had, and so far it's lasted ten years.'

Feresteh tells me about a recurring dream that's been troubling her.

'I think it's because of the drugs they pumped into me in ITU,' she says, tentatively shifting her position in the bed so she's more upright against the pillows. Her face looks scooped, her eyes preternaturally large. 'I was very ill,' she says.

'I'm sorry to hear that.'

'But you know the worst thing about it all is the dream. It comes to me most nights, even sometimes during the day if I sleep a little. It is always the same thing. I am in the hold of sailing ship, with hundreds of girls all my age. And I realise I am being trafficked, about to be taken away across the sea to some faraway place, a place no-one will ever be able to find me. There are heavy pieces of furniture there, too, gaudy, richly decorated. And I come to see that this is how they intend to smuggle us out of the ship – inside the furniture, locked in the chests and the cabinets. I see my father and my uncle looking down at me from the hatch, silhouetted against the light. I call out to them but all they do is wave sadly, and withdraw, and the hatch slides shut, and everything goes quiet. And then the worst thing. From out of the darkness comes a big blue owl. It flies low over our heads, its eyes wide – like THIS – its claws out. And it is so terrifying I put my hands up and I say No! NO! And if I am lucky, I wake up.'

She raises her chin to track the invisible bird, her left arm straight with the fingers of that hand spread, the right arm bent so the hand is level with her face. Her mouth is slightly parted, her breath coming quickly, and her eyes – her eyes are shining.

5: Downtime

The nurses are busy catching up on admin, chatting about this and that, their day, their troubles, their plans. The conversation turns to holidays.

'We were supposed to go to Turkey again this year. Turkey's lovely. Have you been?'

'Yeah. Hot and cheap and that's how I like it.'

'Cornwall's nice but you end up spending just as much, you can't fly there and – let's be honest – it doesn't matter how much you dress it up, the North Atlantic's not the Aegean.'

'Yeah. You go snorkelling and all you'll see are jellyfish and tampons.'

They swap info on some patients, visits and so on, then get back to the important stuff.

'Have you ever been to Egypt?'

'Once.'

'What did you think?'

'It was great. Well I enjoyed it. We stayed on a resort. Sharm El Sheikh. Before the trouble, of course. Everything was controlled on the resort, so you were pretty well looked after. It can get a bit much, getting swamped with demands for money or crappy souvenirs when you go out of the resort into some of the markets. But once you get used to just smiling and saying No thanks they get the message. I told Steve, I said Steve, don't keep waving your hands and saying Maybe later like that. They remember this stuff and bother you worse next time. But he wouldn't have it. It was like he couldn't help himself. And I tell you another weird thing. Steve has a phobia about camels.'

'Camels? Why? Did he get bitten by one or something?'

'No. He'd never seen one before. Just didn't take to them, really. He said it was the way they look at him.'

'Well maybe in retrospect Egypt wasn't a great choice, then. I mean – that's pretty much where all the camels live. Isn't it? I'm right, aren't I?'

'I suppose. Anyway – what happened was, we decided to leave the resort and go to a shop on the outskirts. We wanted to get a lilo and some flip flops, and we thought it'd be a bit cheaper. On the road out to it there's this guy sitting on a camp stool with a big old camel next to him. And of course the man gets up and starts gesturing to the camel, trying to sell us a ride. Steve goes all funny. Keep that thing away from me he says. And he starts walking really quickly to the shop, and I have to make apology faces to the man, and then catch up. So we're in the shop, and I'm having a nose around. I find some flip flops and I turn round to Steve to see what he thinks. And he's not there. So I think – what the hell? And I look out the shop window, and there he is, sitting on top of the camel, with the man standing next to him holding the reins about to set off. So I run out there and I shout Steve! Steve! What the hell are you doing? And it was then I notice the man is wearing Steve's sunglasses. So I ask the man if he'd mind letting Steve down, which he does, eventually. And I get the sunglasses off him, and we walk back to the shop. And I say to Steve, What was that all about? And do you know what he says?'

'I cannot imagine.'

'He says the camel made him do it.'

'The camel?'

'Yep. He said he could see it looking at him through the shop window, and there wasn't a thing he could do about it.'

I tell my opposite number, Aleksy, that I've applied for another job.

'What job?' he says.

'Kind of a counsellor. Using CBT. It comes with a year's post-grad training, so it'd be an amazing opportunity. There's no way I could afford to do it privately.'

He frowns at me steadily.

'You want to do this job?'

'Yeah. I think so.'

'Isn't it a bit – how do you call it? – conceited?'

'How d'you mean, conceited?'

'Well...'

He puts his head on one side, spreads his hands.

'You have problem. You come to me with this problem. I tell you how to solve problem. Because I know best.'

'Maybe. I suppose it's more that you learn some techniques to help the patient break out of unhelpful thought patterns. That's the idea, anyway. You work on finding a solution to the problem together.'

'Hmmm,' says Aleksy. 'I'm not so sure.'

'It's not for everyone.'

'No. That's true. You know – one time – a long time ago now – I was feeling a bit difficult, y'know? So I went to this counsellor. And we sat around in chairs talking. Or at least, I did a lot of talking. Until I thought – what am I doing? Coming here to this place, talking to complete stranger, someone I don't even know? So I stop going, and I sort problem out myself.'

'Fair enough. Like I say, it's not for everyone. It's just one way of addressing a mental health issue. There are others.'

'I went to monastery,' says Aleksy.

'Did you? Wow! A monastery!'

'Why you say wow? What so wow about monastery?'

'Nothing – it's just – it sounds great.'

He shrugs.

'Well. It wasn't like I was there for years. Just one month. I spent long hours going into my head.'

'Meditation.'

'Yes. Meditation. Because there was this lot of noise in my head. It took long time to clean it all out.'

'I've been using a meditation app.'

'An app? What app?'

'Headspace. You get these guided meditations.'

'And you do this every day?'

'Every day. For ten minutes.'

'Is not enough. Ten minutes is not enough. When do you find the time?'

'In the lunch break. I put my sunglasses on and sit in the car. People think I'm just zoning out listening to music.'

'Is not enough. Ten minutes wouldn't even begin to do it for me.'

'You can do longer. I just always seem to stick at ten.'

'I have so much noise in there,' he says, winding his hand in the space above his head. 'There is such a lot of fuss. Ten minutes wouldn't do anything.'

'Maybe I'll try longer.'

'You could join monastery like me.'

'I'd love to.'

And it's true. I would.

I can imagine Aleksy as a monk. With his shaven head, steady gaze, deliberate movements, his economy of being. I can imagine the monastery, high in the mountains. Attacked by warriors in the moonlight. Aleksy deflecting spears with balletic moves, bodies falling like leaves from the cell window. Aleksy calmly putting on a cloak, wandering the desert in search of justice.

'Send me the link,' I say.

Jan is chatting to the care coordinator about her patchy dating history.

'I've kissed my fair share of frogs,' she says. 'Frogs. Trolls. You name it. A whole long line. One guy I saw had one and a half ears.'

'On the same side of his head.'

'He looked alright but he wasn't the kind of guy I normally date. I just didn't fancy him. Not 'cos of the ear thing. I didn't notice the ear thing till the fourth date.'

'You made it to four dates?'

'Yeah – well – it was a slow month.'

'So – what? On the fourth date you asked him back to your place, ran your fingers through his ears, and that was that?'

'We didn't get that far. I only noticed the ear thing when he turned to get his coat. And anyway – even if he had told me I wouldn't have believed him. When we met on the first date, I asked him what he did and he said he was a dust man.'

'A dust man?'

'Yeah. Why? What?'

'I dunno. Dust man sounds odd.'

'Refuse collector, then.'

'Thank you.'

'Anyway. I didn't care what he did, so long as we got on. Only in his case, we didn't.'

'Shame.'

'But you know what he said on the fourth date?'

'What?'

'He said he wasn't really a dust man.'

'What was he, then?'

'He said he was a financial adviser. He said he only told me he was a dust man to check I wasn't going out with him for his money.'

'Tosser.'

'That's what I said.'

'Still. I don't think that's any reason to bite his ear off.'

'Phew! I can't tell you how relieved I am to get that essay out of the way!' says Rachel, dropping an armful of files and folders on to the desk next to me and then herself into the chair. 'It took me right back to when I started uni. And not in a good way.'

'Writing essays is a pain'

'I just find it so stressful. But there! It's done. One good thing though is it reminded me of Mellie, and I haven't thought about her in ages. I wonder what she's doing now?'

'Who's Mellie?'

'She was great. Odd, but great. And I could never quite figure her out, whether she knew she was being odd, or she just was.'

'It's hard to know sometimes.'

'Our first day, the tutor told us to introduce ourselves with our name and then one interesting fact.'

'I hate that.'

'Yeah. Me too. I think I said something lame about how I fell off my skateboard and knocked myself out when I was ten. And that was pretty much how it went round the circle till we got to Mellie. After this strange little pause she always did, y'know? It always put you slightly on edge. So after one of these little pauses she said, really quietly, I've got a dog. And then there was this silence. So eventually the tutor said: And what's your dog called, Mellie? And she said Jism.'

'Jism?'

'I know!'

'That's great! Mind you – there's a teacher at Jess' school called Mr Chisholm.'

'Euch! You'd change your name, wouldn't you?'

'What to?'

'I don't know. Spunkmeyer? Anyway. That's what Mellie was like. We did this session on diabetes once. An introductory thing, looking at the equipment and stuff, and the tutor held up the blood sugar machine and said What would you tell the patient if you had a reading that just said High? So Mellie put up her hand. Yes. Mellie. What would you say? And Mellie put her head on one side, like she was doing an impression of someone being sympathetic, and said I'm sorry to have to tell you but you've got diabetes.'

'That's hilarious.'

'You just couldn't figure out if she was being serious or not. The worst thing time was when we were taking the psychiatric module. We had this tutor who was completely insane. I mean – my god! She always looked as if she was on the edge of something – y'know? Her hair out here, her eyes...'. Rachel widens her eyes, twists her mouth and leans towards me. 'Her hands in her pockets. Anyway, she completely terrified us. And she had this trigger-light temper, and anything would throw her into a rage. Anyway, she'd set us some reading to do, some incredibly heavyweight and tedious article about something or other, and we'd all been out that night and no-one had read it. That session we were all sitting in the classroom, and she started asking us questions about the article. And it was obvious really quickly that no-one had read it. So instead of moving on or making some general comment about how disappointed she was or how important it was to keep up with the reading that she set, she started to make this big personal deal, going round the whole room to see who had read it or not. Everyone said no and looked away, because the more people she asked the more furious she got, until I really thought she'd explode. Then she got to Mellie. And what about you? she said to her, fumbling in her pocket like she'd got a knife in there or something. Did you read my article? So Mellie paused like she used to with everything, looking a bit vacant, and then she said Yes, I did. Oh? said the tutor. I see! Finally! At least one person had the common courtesy to do as I asked. And she was about to move on, but then she stopped, and turned back to Mellie. And what did you find most interesting about my article? she said. And we were all willing her to say something smart. But instead she put her head on the side like she did in diabetes, and she said The end?'

'That's great!'

'A legend!'

'I wonder what she's doing now?'

'Last I heard, she was working in intensive care. Which is something else. I mean – imagine coming out of your coma and seeing Mellie leaning over you with her head on one side. *God* knows what she'd say...'

Ethan's one our most experienced nurses, with a background in so many areas of acute medicine –A&E, ITU and so on – he's definitely earned his stripes. He's talking about the different infections and things he saw when he worked in Sexual Health, illustrating each dreadful detail with a vaudevillian relish, raising his eyebrows, staring at you for a second with wide eyes, then dropping his jaw, rocking back in the chair and laughing energetically.

'The Sexual Health Clinic was great fun,' he says, one leg crooked over the other, idly tracing the arched line of his eyebrow with a fingernail. 'I saw some pretty weird things there, I can tell you. There's this thing called Trichomonas vaginalis. It's an 'orrible little protozoan parasite that lives in the vaginal tract or the urethra. Men can get it but it's mostly women. Anyway, it's proper disgusting. Shaped like a pear with these flagella whipping about. Lives on scraps of dead cells, runs around causing infection. I saw one under the microscope. It looked happy enough, though, swimming around on the slide. I think it actually saw me.' And holding on to the back of the chair with one hand, he suddenly tips back, sticks his legs out and kicks them like he's doing the backstroke at the pool, waving up at himself looking down through the lens of the microscope. 'Coo ee!' he says. Then he straightens again. 'I don't know. We had one woman come in. She said she knew she had a dose and had been trying to cure herself.'

'I hate to ask – but – how?'

'She'd been rubbing her fanny with raw hamburger. You know – to tempt them out. To tempt them out!'

He stares at me for a second, then laughs.

'It's true!' he screams. 'Honest to God! I'm laughing, but it's true!'

Two nurses chat in the queue for the photocopier.

'I went on that dating app you told me about.'

'Yeah? How d'you get on?'

'Alright. I struggled a bit with my profile. I thought I sounded a bit boring, so when it said hobbies, I put chess.'

'Chess?'

'Yeah. Why?'

'Can you even play chess?'

'No.'

'Aren't you worried you'll get found out?'

'We're hardly likely to be playing chess on our first date, are we? Unless they're a complete perv.'

'But what if they ask you about it?'

'I'll just say I like to play it now and again and that's it.'

'But what if they ask you stuff?'

'Like what?'

'I don't know. Who your favourite player is.'

'They won't.'

'Don't you think it might put them off?'

'I've already had two dates.'

'Two?'

'Two.'

'They must be desperate.'

'Thanks a lot.'

(We all move up a spot)

'Oh yeah. I know what I wanted to tell you. I was at the doctor's the other day and there's this kid with his hoodie up standing in front of me in the queue, shuffling about. And I think to myself – hang on a minute, that's Tiffany's youngest, Brandon. So I tap him on the shoulder, and he turns round, and fuck me, it was! So I says to him "What are you doing here, Brandon?" – but then I think – No! Noooo no no! That's naughty. I can't be asking him that. I mean, he might go and tell me, and that'd be awkward. For both of us. I mean – I'm best mates with Tiffany and I might struggle not to spill the beans. But do you know what he says? He says "I'm too embarrassed." So I say "Well you gotta tell me now." And he goes: "No. You'll just think I'm a dullard."

'A dullard?'

'A dullard. That's what he says. A dullard. I didn't even know what it meant. I thought it was some kind of duck.'

'What teenage boy uses a word like dullard?'

'A Brandon-type boy, obviously Shell. Anyway, I say to him:

"Whatever it is I won't think any the worse of you. Promise." So he says: "I've got a fingernail stuck in my throat"'.

'A fingernail?'

'He bites his nails and swallows it. And a bit got stuck in his throat.'

'Urgh! Who bites their nails and swallows it? Gack!'

'Yeah? Well – sorry to ruin your world, Shell, but a lot of people do. And not everyone who picks their nose flicks it, neither.'

'That's got to be one of the worst discharges I've ever had the displeasure of seeing. I mean – for heaven's sake! It was tantamount to fly-tipping!'

Rosie is smiling like she always does – an easy, enfolding, wise-woman kind of smile that's been tested for years in the community and is all the warmer for it – but I can tell even Rosie is shocked.

'I mean – poor thing's end stage COPD. Thin as a rake. Can't stand on her own – certainly not safely. I wouldn't send her home with a live-in carer, but she's still only got people going in twice a day. When I went in, she wasn't wearing her nasal specs, so her SATS were non-existent. She was in a right state.'

'So what did you do?'

'I sent her straight back in! I know they're short of beds, but that was ridiculous.'

It's early evening. The rapid response office is cooler and calmer. The change from the morning is astonishing. Then, every desk space was occupied, the kitchen crowded with people making drinks, people walking backwards and forwards, stopping for urgent briefings, catching-up, gossiping, serious conversations, hilarious conversations, secretive conversations, the whole thing layering and building and rising with the press of the day's business until it reaches a peak and all you hear is a great massy buzz, the murmuration of a large community health team getting ready to fly out over the city. Now, at the end of the day, the last of us are coming back, handing over, doing admin. It's quiet. There's plenty of space. I love it.

'And that's not all,' says Rosie, sitting on the edge of the desk and reaching into her pocket. 'I brought back a friend...'

She pulls out a clear plastic specimen tube, about as big as your thumb, with a screw-top lid. She holds it in front of her and gives it a little shake. Inside is a bed bug. It's on its back wiggling its legs in the air, but she taps the tube helpfully, it rights itself, and begins pacing up and down the tube, exploring the confines of its prison.

'The place was riddled,' she says. 'They were supposed to have fumigated it, but it obviously didn't work. You'd think they'd have checked. These things are indestructible.'

She waggles the tube again; the bed bug tenses.

'I heard they're a really ancient life form. They were being a pain when the dinosaurs were around. Although they probably weren't called bed bugs then.'

'No? Probably tyrannosaurus rex bugs.'

'Bronto bugs.'

'Jurassic pain in the arse bugs.'

One of the admin workers at the far end of the office has the radio on quietly, which is always a nice touch this time of day. It starts to play the famous intro to that Frank Sinatra song, New York, New York.

Rosie gives the tube another shake and holds it up to her face to have a close look.

'They're quite cute, in a horrible kind of way,' she says. 'I suppose we've all got our roles in life. You have to respect that.'

'What are you going to do with it?'

'Oh – I thought I'd probably put him down the toilet. Burial at sea. Poor thing. I've got enough pets, though.'

She smiles, and starts singing along with Frank.

'I'll make a brand new start of it, New Yoooork, New Yoooork...'

She slips the tube back in her pocket and jumps off the desk.

'But that's the way of the world, I guess. Somebody singing New York, New York, somebody getting flushed.'

❧

Rachel brings her tea over and sits with me.

'What've you been up to?' I ask her.

'House hunting,' she says.

'How's that going?'

'Terrible. I had the worst day the other day. I saw nine houses.'

'Nine?'

'I know. I just booked out the entire morning and went.'

'Did Ben go?'

'Ben? No! He can't stand it. But you play to your strengths. I'm what you might call the triage nurse in this relationship, especially as far as houses go. I sift out the crap. Which is all of them.'

'It's a thing, that's for sure.'

'I had the weirdest estate agent show me round. She was only young. About twenty, I'd guess, her hair all piled up. And she had this heavy makeup that stopped at her chin, circling her features, which made her look a bit like a giant egg. I couldn't help asking about it. I do it like that so I don't get raped she said'

'What a thing to say!'

'I know! She was wearing this extraordinary outfit. White fur jacket split at the sides, bright pantaloon trousers and leather boots. Although she was barefoot when I met her at the office. She was sitting on a chair digging her toes into the carpet. Mmm she said. Feel that!'

'Weird!'

'That's not the half of it. When we got into the car she said she knew right off we'd get along because she gets a feeling about people. She said she thought I was a florist, and when I said I was a nurse, she said yeah, I'm not surprised, because you totally look like one. And anyway, she said, I'm just glad you're not like the usual stiffs I have to show round.'

'Wow!'

'And then there were the houses. Honestly, Jim – it was like we were scouting sets for a horror film. The first one was a bungalow right the other side of town, down by the river. I mean literally by the river. On the flood plain. Don't worry, she said. It only floods when it's tidal.

What – you mean like twice a day? I said. You're up some steps so you're good, she said. Anyway, it's an unadopted road, which people love. It means you can do what you want with it. I reckon it's more that the council know it floods and have washed their hands, I said, but she ignored that and showed me round. A dismal, lightless hole that should've been condemned, let alone put on the market. No? she said – okay – I'll show you some more.

The next one was worse. It had this terrible atmosphere, creepy and sad, like someone had died or been murdered. I asked her if anyone was living there at the moment because I couldn't tell. There was a mattress on the floor, and the sheets were thrown back, odd things scattered about. She said yeah, a woman and her kid. She's getting divorced or something. Honestly, Jim – I wanted to start taking some details so I could call social services. I mean – it was getting a bit too much like being at work. Anyway, that was no good, so we drove over to the next house and out of the blue she asked me if liked macaroni cheese? I said yep, love it. I said we're vegetarian, so we have macaroni cheese a lot. Have you tried it with bacon on the top? she said, because that is the absolute nuts. And I said well...no, because we're vegetarian. So she said shame, so maybe just a bit of ham, then?

The next house she showed me had an enormous crack right down the middle. I mean huge, like if you slammed the door it would fall apart in two halves. Oh that? she said. That's just subsidence. I sold a house exactly like this the other day for four-fifty. Then she laughed and said There's no way they'll be able to resell. I wanted to say to her – you do know that's not a good story to be telling me in this situation, right? But what was the point?

The last house she showed me belonged to this elderly guy. The estate agent stayed outside stomping up and down having some huge argument on her phone whilst the guy showed me round. It was run-down, like all the others, but of course I was going through the rooms making lots of encouraging noises like you do. Oh – I love what you've done in the bathroom. Those brown tiles are really so, I don't know, quirky – kind of thing. He was right up close behind me the whole time, breathing down my neck, which was unnerving. Every time I turned round he was there, smiling with his neck stretched out like a tortoise. I went into the bedroom and there was an enormous cactus in a pot. I mean gigantic – the same height as me. I turned round and there he was, smiling away. I can see you approve of my phallic cactus he said, licking his lips. And that's when the estate agent came in. What d'you think, she said, clapping her hands. Sold?'

We were talking about difficult neighbours we'd had to put up with over the years.

'First time we moved to Bristol, we rented a couple of rooms in Bedminster. It was alright, except the bathroom was out on the landing and we had to share it with the flat downstairs. Kind of a bedsit, really, come to think about it. Anyway, the couple downstairs were difficult. They were both drinkers. She was a nervous type – pale and trembly, eyeliner and lipstick all over the place like she'd done it on a trampoline. Her husband was the worst, though. He looked like he was made out of tyres, love and hate on his knuckles, bike chain round his neck. They used to sleep all day, go out, then come back and fight. One night I was in the bathroom getting ready for bed and I heard them come in. She stood at the bottom of the stairs, saw the light on, and screamed: I am NOT using the bucket again.'

'Classy.'

'We moved out pretty quick.'

'I shared a flat with this guy once. Gavin. He was lovely. Bit of a stoner. He was a self-employed gardener. An expert on wisteria – so he said, anyway. He used to come home, throw his receipts under the bed, put The Fall on the record player and we'd smoke skunk all night, staring into the fire and laughing. It was lovely. Then he crashed his bike and fell in love with the nurse who stopped to help. She moved in the next week and took over. She had this thing about crocheting bags with string. I came down to breakfast and there were hundreds of little crochet string bags hanging everywhere, a bulb of garlic in one, half a lemon in another. And she really started to freeze me out, too, like she wanted Gavin all for herself. I had this nightmare where I got wrapped in a big string bag by a giant spider in a nurse's uniform. Anyway – in the end they sat me down and had the conversation. Shame. I liked living with Gavin.'

'Yeah? Well – we lived next door to this couple. Young professionals. I can't remember what he did, but she was something in travel. She was really into magic eggs.'

'Wha'd'ya mean, magic eggs?'

'Eggs. You know. Made of crystal. You power them up with psychic energy, and then use them for healing and protection and whatnot. It's that bullshit thing where you hold out your arm and ask someone to push it down – which they easily do – and then you hold an egg in your hand, and ask them to try again, and they can't? You get different sizes of egg, depending on the job. I never believed it – although I thought maybe I might benefit from some overflow egg power, because we were living right next door, and the auras aren't password protected, are they? Anyway, she was nice enough. We went out for drinks a couple of times. It was all good. But a couple of months later we came back and there was this letter waiting for us, pushed under the door. It was written in a real psycho font – y'know? – shaky green sentences, wandering all over.'

'Saying what?'

'Saying how she was sorry for thinking all these bad things about me, apologising for all the things she'd done.'

'Like what?'

'I couldn't make it out. But the page was covered in it. And then worst of all, there was a clump of hair in with the letter.'

'Euch! What did you do?'

'We went round. It was all dark, so we thought maybe they were out. But we knocked anyway and after a minute he came to the door. We showed him the letter, and said as gently as we could that we were a bit worried about her, and was she okay and everything.'

'What did he say?'

'That was the other weird thing. He didn't seem particularly surprised or fazed about it. He just kinda waved it in the air and said: Ah – yeah! The letters! – and that was it. We saw her a couple of times after that and it was like nothing happened. We didn't bring it up again, and moved a few months later.'

'Sounds like it might've been a regular thing.'

'Yeah. Bad eggs. Who knows? I never did experience the power myself. But then again, apparently you have to wear a special receiver on your head to really get the benefit.'

A couple of the nurses are sitting with the Co-ordinator, chatting about this and that at the end of the shift.

'I'm sure that house is haunted' says Lena. 'Every time I go there something weird happens.'

'Like what?'

'I don't know. Just weird. Like – atmospheres or something.'

'My mum and dad had a poltergeist for a while,' says Rachel, flipping through a file, so matter-of-fact it's like she's just turning to a section called Paranormal Manifestations and What to Do About Them.

'What d'you mean for a while? Did they have it exorcised?'

'Not really. We got to the bottom of it ourselves.'

'So what happened?'

'Well – they sold up and moved to this spooky new house on Bodmin Moor. It used to be the parrot house of a big old stately home...'

'The Parrot house?'

'Where they used to keep parrots.'

'Makes sense'

'It's pretty isolated. Just the main house which is all converted into flats now. A few outbuildings. And then the parrot house, standing on its own at the edge of the land. And then beyond that, you've got the moors, stretching out all bleak and mysterious, with a load of sheep and goats grazing and generally wandering about.'

'Why the hell'd they go there?'

'They wanted to get away from it all.'

'Sounds like they did.'

'Absolutely. It's nice enough when the sun's shining. Anyway – they said to me the place was lovely and everything but might be a little bit haunted. So I said fine, I'll have a look. The first night, everything was quiet, fine, nothing strange about it except for those creaky noises you always get in old houses.'

'I hate them.'

'But the following morning when we all came down to breakfast, the heavy rug in the front room was pushed all the way over to one side, rucked up against the sofa.'

'That's what gets me about ghosts. They never do anything constructive. Hundreds of years to plan their revenge or whatever, and all they end up doing is arsing around with the furniture.'

'Yeah – but turns out, this wasn't a ghost. It was just a static charge building up between the rug and the stone flags, so overnight it kind of floated across the floor. We put some anti-static strips down, and it sorted it out a treat.'

Nice.'

'The second night was different though. We'd all sat down to watch Strictly, when suddenly the television shot across the room and smashed against the wall'

'Oh my God! That's terrifying! You can't tell me that was static.'

'No. Turns out the aerial was hanging loose outside, a goat caught his horn in it and dragged the TV across the room when he tried to run off.'

We're standing back at Magda's car, wondering what to do next. I've just noticed her hair, cut for the New Year. Shaved close up one side, the rest in a heavy blonde fringe she continually scoots out of her face. She looks tired but I don't say it.

Magda is the hardest working person I know. Not only does she pull extra shifts as a nursing assistant, but she works most weekend nights as door security on the clubs and bars in the city. I'm guessing she hasn't slept in three days.

'Man,' she says. 'I don't think I can do this anymore. It's not worth it.'

'Why? What happened?'

'Do you ever get those nights when you think – shit! Did I miss something? Did they fly a plane over town and pump it full of crazy spray?'

'Did you get some trouble, then?'

'Did I get some trouble? Yes, I got some trouble, thank you very much for asking. The funny thing was, they put me on the door of that comedy club you were talking about the other day. And I was thinking – okay, my only trouble here will be staying awake. But then these four guys show up, enormous guys, the kinds of guys who play rugby or some such shit, and I don't know, bend girders for living. Gigantic pain in the arse kinda guys. And when they turn up to the club they're already pretty drunk. So I say to the bar manager, I say to him: Watch those guys and don't sell them any more beer if they start getting too loud, y'know what I'm saying? They've already had too much. But of course, what do they do? They sell them plenty. And the next thing you know they start getting very loud and very aggressive, particularly this one guy, the biggest and tallest. So I go over to him, and I lay my hand on his shoulder like this, and I say to him: Can I ask you to please keep it down? Otherwise you'll be asked to leave. And you know what he says to me?'

'No. What does he say?'

'He says fuck you.'

'Wow.'

'I tell you, man, I was like: Don't you be saying fuck you to me! Who the fuck do you think you are, saying fuck you to me? And his friends are like: We're very sorry. It's his birthday. And I say I don't care if it's he just won the Nobel prize for fucking CHEMISTRY. There's no call to be so nasty to me. And then the other guys stand in front of him and they say: It's just the beer. He's not normally like this. He's normally kind and quiet and basically a mouse. And I say: Well I'm sorry to have to tell you, but it's not the beer making him a dickhead. The beer is absolutely fine. It's your friend being a dickhead that makes him a dickhead. And the guy leans through them, and he says to me: Hey! You! You're much too pretty to be doing a job like this. So I say to him: Keep your sexist opinions to yourself, my friend or you'll see what this pretty girl's capable of. Meanwhile all his stupid friends are crowding round saying sorry, sorry, sorry, please forgive him. And then the guy himself starts saying sorry, putting his hands together doing a pisshead kind of namaste. So I said: Okay. Okay. Against my better judgement, and because it's your birthday, I'm gonna give you one last chance. And they're all like thank you, oh thank you very much and everything. And I'm just about to go when I give the guy one last look and you know what he does? He flips me the middle finger. That's it. I don't wait for backup. I'm too mad and I'm too tired. I just grab him by the collar and march him out. And all his friends are jumping up and down saying sorry and he won't do it again and please don't, it's his birthday. And you know what I say?'

'What?'

'I say Happy Birthday, Dickhead. Now fuck off and don't come back.'

She sweeps her hair back from her face and takes a long drink of tea.

With her large round eyes, accentuated with dark blue-black eyeshadow and heavy black mascara, her pale face, and her sleepy demeanour, she reminds me of a panda. But even though Magda is a good friend of mine, and she's used to seeing me around, still, I wouldn't fancy getting on the wrong side of her. No way would I rile her up. I've seen how she crunches bamboo; I've seen what she can do with those paws.

As soon as I've claimed a workspace with my bag I head for the kitchen. The kitchen is always the best place to start in the morning. It's a watering hole, a place of mutual support, commiseration, inspiration, the first place to get the measure of the day. And coffee.

I've come in midway through a conversation between Gemma, the OT, and Faith, one of the bank nurses.

Gemma's pregnant. Very pregnant. In fact, Gemma is SO pregnant, she gets asked a dozen times a day how much longer she plans coming in, as if the questioner thinks she's slightly unhinged, and they're worried they're going to find her conducting a patient assessment with a bloody baby bumping along behind her, desperately trying to gum its way free of the cord.

'…because you really are so big and out front,' says Faith, stirring her hot chocolate slowly, before licking the spoon and then using it to trace in the air the generous outline of Gemma's belly. 'I imagine this means you will be having another boy.'

'I don't think so,' says Gemma, leaning back against the sink, looking a little flushed despite the early hour. 'The scan was pretty clearly a girl. But I'd be happy either way.'

'Ah – you see! But these scans and things, they can be wrong. I had a friend back in Zimbabwe, she was forty-two years of age, and she had one more baby, and she decided enough was enough. So when the baby came she called him Finish, and she went straightaway and had her tubes tied. But then, you see, the next year, because of recanalization or something else I don't know what – the very next year, she fell pregnant again. And she gave birth to a healthy baby girl. And do you know what they call this baby girl?'

'Miracle?'

'No. But that would have been a good name. No! They call this baby girl Stop!'

'What were her middle names? Please, Dear and God?'

'I don't know that she had any middle names. No – it was just Stop, I think. So then she went back to the surgeon, and he said okay,okay, and he tied the tubes a little tighter this time, and that was that. Six children, and hardly room to put four.'

'I'd be happy with three. I think three's plenty.'

'Yes. Three is a good number.'

Faith picks up her hot chocolate, takes a sip, then cradles it ruminatively beneath her chin.

'But you know something, Gemma – I can NOT think of anything in nature with three of anything. Can you? Four legs on an elephant. Four legs on a cat. Two on a kangaroo. But three…?'

'I think an octopus has three hearts,' I say, squeezing in between them to get some hot water from the kettle.

'Ah! Well! There you go, then,' says Faith, laughing. 'You wouldn't want to be like an octopus, would you, Gemma? Although, maybe that wouldn't be such a bad idea. That's one thing you definitely need more of with babies.'

'What – hearts?'

'Arms.'

6: Running on Empty

The front door is open. When I go in and close it, I see a sign thumb-tacked just above the letter box: Keep The Door Closed.

I can hear Raymond talking animatedly on the phone in the front room. When I stick my head round the corner and wave, he waggles his free hand in the air and continues:

'This is absolutely fucking ridiculous.... of course I can't tell you the card number... well, for the simple reason I've lost the card. That's the entire purpose of my call. If I had the card to read the number I wouldn't be ringing you, would I? No I won't calm down. I demand that you reinstate the two hundred pounds that was stolen from my account.... I don't KNOW how they got the pin number. They're CRIMINALS. That's their JOB. All I want is for you to do YOUR job and give me back my money....'

Something happens with the phone. He curses, holds it away from his face, bangs it twice on the arm of the chair and then tosses it out into the chaos of the room.

'Battery's dead!' he says. 'You couldn't do me a favour, could you?'

'Of course.'

'Locate the base that's somewhere over there and charge it up again?'

The little front room is in a mess, as devastating as if flood water had unexpectedly rushed through the house and then back out again, leaving a tangled tideline of random stuff – trainers, trousers, duvet covers, exercise bike, milk cartons, who knows what. The only clarity in the place are the bookshelves, safely screwed to the walls out of harm's way, the books neatly aligned in height order. They mostly seem to be about film, especially animation. Which makes sense, given the display on the hallway wall of some early Disney drawings –

character studies of Jiminy Cricket, Figaro the cat, Pinocchio.

I'd had some warning of the state of play this morning. The therapist who'd been in to see Raymond the day before had written an illuminating note: Patient reports that a stranger visited last night with a bottle of brandy – stayed for sex – stole money on his card. Police informed.

Notes further back show that this isn't an unusual event. Raymond has a long history of alcohol abuse and all the associated complications, medical and social. I've come round to dress the wound on his head, and generally see how he's doing.

He has no recollection of the fall.

'Is that unusual for you?' I say, gently cleaning the wound with saline, holding a swab to his eyeline to catch the drips.

'No, sadly,' he says. 'It's the booze, of course.'

'I read that you tried a detox programme last year – which is good.'

'Is it? Well – you get shunted into these things. My heart wasn't in it. I'm afraid I didn't just fall off the wagon I rolled it over and took everyone down with me.'

'Worth trying again...?'

'I don't think so,' he says, with a deflationary sigh.

I photograph the wound, dress it, check him over more thoroughly. He's got lots of injuries, old bruises, new bruises. It's like he drinks a bottle of brandy then throws himself into a giant tumbling machine. It's a miracle he ever emerges.

'I love the Disney drawings you have on the wall,' I say.

'Thank you.'

'I remember the first time I saw Pinocchio. That scene where Lampy turns into a donkey. Good grief! And that bit where Pinocchio's walking on the seabed with a rock tied to his tail. Calling out Faaaa...tttthhhherrr! And all the seahorses and clams and things come out to look. But when he asks them if they've seen Monstro the whale, they look terrified and disappear! I mean – what an absolute freakin' nightmare!'

'Yes,' says Raymond. 'I know. Story of my life.'

Despite having to work in an office that looks suspiciously like a converted cupboard, Alice, the warden is remarkably upbeat.

'Have you come to see Terry?' she says, squeezing past a heap of junk out into the hostel landing. 'Shall I show you the way? It's a bit of a warren...'

Even though I have been before, I know how confusing the layout is, so I say 'That'd be great, thanks.'

'Poor old Terry,' she says, locking the cupboard/office door behind her then marching off up a set of stairs so narrowly twisting and creaking it's like being processed the wrong way through the guts of a dilapidated monster. 'He's had such a time of it. We're a bit worried about him, to be honest. He's wasting away. I mean – he barely eats a thing, and he's not going out like he used to. Mind you...' she says, pushing through a fire door and then on through a series of branching corridors, '...at least he's not seeing Keith.' She turns and frowns at me, as if to say You know – KEITH, then carries on down the corridor. I feel like I'm in one of those nightmares where the way gets smaller and smaller and you end up on your knees tapping with one finger on a door the size of your hand. But suddenly Alice stops, turns on the spot, raps smartly on the door to her left, and goes in.

She's right about Terry wasting away. What makes his condition worse, somehow, is the contrast between his emaciated body and the dark luxuriance of his beard and hair, curling upwards and outwards with such vigour you'd think they were wigs, stuck on a cadaver for the contrast. Terry's still in his green hospital pyjamas, an ID band around his wrist. It says in the notes he self-discharged, against advice. Quite how he made it home I've no idea, although maybe Keith helped.

The room is a mess. Someone has had a rudimentary go at clearing some space at least, the piles of trash and bags and boxes and clothes pushed to one side of the room, occupying every spare foot of the galley kitchen surfaces and sink, giving the bedsit a lopsided feel. A light breeze plays in from the sea just a fag-flick away through the window, dispelling to some extent the heavy atmosphere in the room.

'Sorry it's in such a two-and-eight,' says Terry, struggling to sit up on the edge of his soiled bed and then picking at his nails. 'I haven't had a chance to tidy up.'

'We'll get it sorted, Terry,' says Alice. 'Anyway. Listen. There's a support worker guy coming later with some supplies. So that's good.' She pauses a moment, raising her eyebrows and smiling, to let the good news percolate through, I suppose. Terry waves his hand; she nods emphatically again. ''Okay! I'll leave you to it, then,' she whispers, and quietly closes the door behind her.

'Diamond girl, Alice,' says Terry. 'They all are.'

'I like their office.'

'It's a cupboard.'

'I thought so.'

'They 'ain't got no money for nuthin'.'

'No. I guess not.'

'They do their best though.'

I'm halfway through the exam when there's another knock on the door and Jack, the support worker steps inside. Jack's enormous, a bear in a parka, check shirt and caterpillar boots, holding a carrier bag of shopping in either paw. I say hello. He looks startled to see me there.

'I bought you a selection of things,' he says, eventually. 'Honey nut cornflakes, bread, milk, biscuits, tea. Y'know. The basics. Alice gave me a list.'

'That's kind of you, mate. Thanks,' says Terry. 'I need fattening up.'

Jack looks at him, then at me, then at Terry again, then carries on unpacking. Although it's hardly unpacking – more like stacking – in the one clear corner of the kitchen he can find. He hesitates before opening the fridge to put the milk and butter away, then does it at arm's length.

'There!' he says, closing the fridge again. 'All done! We'll be back this afternoon to talk about some other stuff, but I'll let you crack on for now.'

'Okay mate. Thanks again,' says Terry. Jack clumps out and shuts the door.

'I can't complain,' says Terry, crooking one leg over the other and crossing his arms. 'I 'ain't got no reason not to get better.'

He starts telling me about his recent past. How he fell in with some big-time gangster who let him stay in the cottage in his grounds rent free for a little delivery work.

'Man – you shoulda seen that place!' says Terry. 'The house was like a castle. Actually I think it was a castle. He had this pond in the middle of the lawn, and it was filled with these enormous fish, all floodlit, swimming about like bastards. Each one of 'em worth a monkey. And the cars he had. From little fancy Italian sports jobbies to big fuck-off landrovers, all of 'em in temperature-controlled stables.'

'Didn't have any horses then?'

'Horses? Nah! He didn't like horses. 'Cept down the track. Anyway, one night I was in the cottage, minding my own, having a little puff, when there was all these flashing lights outside, and I know it sounds stupid but at first I thought some'ink had gone wrong with the fish pond. But then it was all like Police! Open up! And I'm like How do I know you're the old bill? Anyone can shout anything. So they smashes the door down and they drag me outside. They were after my mate, 'course. Same old story. They was always trying it on. But they didn't have nothing. He was a lot of things, but he wasn't careless.'

'So then what happened?'

'It all went a bit Pete, I didn't have no scratch, so I split.'

He shrugs, then leans forwards on his folded arms to inspect his leg as it kicks up and down.

'Funny how it goes, innit?'

It's quite a contrast to see the two of them together – Alex, wraith-like, matted hair, scooped eyes, shivering, hugging his legs in bed with a filthy duvet piled up around him; and Graham, the support worker from the alcohol and substance abuse team, shaven-headed, gym-fit, in a smart grey reefer jacket and leather man bag, perched on the arm of the sofa with his hands in his pockets.

'You've got this far, yeah?' says Graham. 'Hats off to you, mate. It's no easy thing you've done there. Don't go and spoil it now. After all we've been through. You got to realise – this is a disease we're talking about, yeah? There are all kindsa toxins and shit floatin' around your body right now. You can't just expect to jump up and be cured. It's a long, hard process. And you're doin' great, man! Isn't he? This guy'll tell ya…'

'You are. Graham's right. Alcohol addiction's the hardest thing.'

'See what I mean?'

Alex doesn't seem convinced. He draws his legs closer to him, gives his head a peremptory shake.

'I don' know, man. I jus' feel like I'm wastin' everyone's time. I mean – I brought it on myself.'

'You can't afford to think like that,' says Graham. 'Everyone's different. You're totally worth it, man.'

'Is there a social worker involved?' I ask Graham, flipping through his folder.

'No,' he says. 'When they see they're still drinking they pull out.'

He shrugs, scuffs his shoes in the trash.

'It's hard, but it's just the way it is.'

'It's not like I'm not trying,' says Alex.

'Yeah – but there's trying, and there's doing, Alex. You've got to be in a position to accept the help. It's just how it works. You know that.'

'Yeah.'

'We're here for you, though.'

There are several bottles within easy reach of Alex's bed – a two litre bottle of cider, a couple of quarter bottles of vodka, some other, less obvious stuff in bottles with the labels torn off. A dull yellow light filters through the filthy windows. The flat is an apocalyptic mess; it looks like an extemporary shelter somebody hollowed out with their hands in a landfill site. Here and there you can just make out traces of the orderly life Alex once used to live. There's a mountain bike in the hallway, quietly fossilising under a press of junk; over by the window-ledge, a toolbox, some work boots.

'We've got to find a way to keep you out of trouble long enough to detox properly,' says Graham. 'Yeah?'

'Yeah,' says Alex. He doesn't sound convinced.

Graham shrugs, pushes his hands deeper into his jacket.

'How long've we known each now?' he says. 'Gotta be nine, ten years.'

'Is it?' says Alex, rubbing his face. 'Fuck, man! Nine years? No! That's like…' He screws up his face to figure out what percentage of his life that represents: '…that's like… a fuck of a long time, man!'

'I think so,' says Graham. 'First time I met you you'd just been beaten up and taken to hospital. You were in a bad way, my friend.'

'Was I?' says Alex. 'I don't remember.'

'Yeah – well – you don't remember much, to be fair. You didn't remember I was here yesterday, so maybe that's not headline news.'

'No. You're right. Probably not.'

'I've seen you in and out of hospital a hundred times. Lost sight of you for months on end when you took yourself off somewhere. You'd always turn up again, half dead, some new injury. And now look.'

He's right. I'm reading through the latest discharge summary. For someone so young, Alex has a terrible list of things wrong. In fact, it's a miracle he's still here at all. Looking at him on the bed, though, it would be easy to think that maybe he wasn't – that maybe he'd died that last time in hospital, but his spirit was so cussed it dragged itself back across town to find rest in this cold, cold bed.

'It's like training, yeah? You can't just jump on a treadmill and bang out ten K. You might feel great at the end of it, but the truth is, if you don't get the intervals right you can be setting yourself up for a lot of trouble. It's all about the interaction between the sympathetic and the parasympathetic nervous systems, the way your body metabolises the shit and tries to get straight again. Jim'll tell you. Hey?'

They both look at me – Graham as if he's about to pick me up and bench press me, Alex with a haunted, shivery look.

'That's right,' I say, 'Uh-huh.'

With his thick black hair shaved at the sides and gelled back in a riotous, rockabilly quiff, white framed sunglasses and perfect designer stubble on perfect designer cheekbones, Ethan the nurse makes every visit a fashion shoot. I can see him waiting for me further up the street. He's lounging back against a lamppost, one white trainer kicked back, the furry grey hood of his parka arrayed like a luxurious ruff around his neck. He's snapping gum, staring at the cars going by. He looks fabulous.

'Oh there you are !' he says, pushing himself upright, flashing me a look over the rim of his sunglasses. 'I wondered where you were. I was clean-shaven when I got 'ere.'

We've come to see Martin, a difficult patient with a history of drug and alcohol abuse, a few incidents of aggression. I've met Martin before – admittedly a while ago. He's young, but only on paper. When I met him, he'd just been discharged from hospital following a fall down a dozen steps and a long lie at the bottom. The fact he survived at all was a miracle. But miracles are fleeting, and there's always something waiting the other side of them. In Martin's case it's a list of medical acronyms that reads like a roll call for the damned. What's worse is his recent history of non-compliance, missed appointments, saying one thing and doing the opposite. He was referred to us by the hospital again, this time to dress an abscess in his thigh, the latest wound from his attempts to find anything resembling a patent vein. We've been formally tasked to get him to sign an official waiver if he declines help again, so long as we feel he has capacity.

'Feeling lucky?' I say to Ethan.

'Darling – I was born lucky,' he says. 'The rest is just exercise and a great skincare routine.'

Martin is staying in supported housing – in this case, a pleasant-looking semi in a tree-lined street, a tall privet hedge screening it off from passers-by. A mosaic path runs from a gap in the hedge through a functional, stone chipped garden to the front door. There's a brushed steel intercom by the door with a line of illegible, rain-smeared names by the buttons.

'Shall we ring it?' says Ethan.

'Let's ring it.'

'You ring it.'

'No you ring it.'

'Okay I'll ring it.'

Ethan rings it.

Rings again.

Eventually a woman answers in a drawly voice.

'Who is it?' she says.

'Oh hi there!' says Ethan, leaning closer to the intercom and giving me a cartoon-panicky look at the same time. 'It's Ethan and Jim, nurses from the rapid response team? We've come to see Martin?'

'He can't see you. He's ill,' she says.

'Ah. Well. That's probably a good reason for us to come in, then. I mean – you know – being nurses and everything...'

'I told you. He's ill. Come back tomorrow.'

'Erm... we kind of need to see him face to face so he can tell us himself,' says Ethan. 'Otherwise we'll get in trouble. Would that be alright?'

'No,' she says. 'Come back tomorrow.'

The intercom goes dead.

Whilst we're standing there wondering what to do next, a man and a dog appear through the hedge. They both look extraordinary – the man because he has a heavily tattooed face and more piercings than the cenobites in Hellraiser; the dog because it has three legs and a lop-sided, piratical expression.

'Who'ya'fter?' he says.

'Oh, hi there!' says Ethan, shrugging and tipping his head

coquettishly on one side. 'We were just wondering if we could come in and see Martin?'

'Martin?' says the man, frowning. 'No. You can't. He's ill.'

'Yeah. I know. We're nurses.'

The man fishes a key out of his pocket (although I wouldn't have been surprised if he pulled it out of his ear).

'No,' he says. 'Come back tomorrow.'

And he lets himself in.

Only the dog looks back.

The door slams shut.

'Fine! Suit yourself!' says Ethan, shouldering his bag. 'Waste my time why don't you!'

He puts his sunglasses back on, and we leave. The sun comes out. Ethan walks down the path with an exaggerated throw of his hips.

'Work it, baby!' he says.

❧

Mandy's flat is at the top of the block – so much so that the lift doesn't extend there, and we have to walk the last two flights. It makes me think of an osprey's nest, a junky bundle of sticks wedged in the uppermost branches of a pine. The nest is made up of old music magazines, Janice Joplin posters, empty cans, unpaid bills, unopened nutritional milkshakes, and the osprey itself is a haggard, featherless old bird, smoking a roll-up, staring unblinking over the city.

'I'm a singer' Mandy says, her voice so broken she can hardly talk. 'Or was. 'scuse the mess.'

She offers us a seat – a dirt-shined cushion in a sixties wicker chair, and a spot at the end of the crapped-up sofa. Standing isn't an option, but at least this is the last job of the day.

'Thanks,' I say, and we both – slowly – sit down.

I hardly know where to start. We'd come to see Mandy as a double-up as the notes on her file described how she'd been hearing evil voices telling her to tear herself and other people up.

'But don't worry. A and E did a risk assessment,' said the co-ordinator. 'No history of violence, and they don't think this was a psychotic episode, as such.'

'As such?'

'No. More to do with alcohol withdrawal. So doubling up should cover it.'

I've never really understood the doubling-up rule. The way I see it, it doesn't matter how many people you send in, someone's going to get hurt. If anything, having other people with you only acts as a distraction. Although it does make me think of that joke about the two rangers walking in the forest, talking about the danger from grizzly bears. 'Because they run pretty fast, you know.' 'Yeah?' says the other. 'Well I don't have to run faster than a grizzly bear, Chuck. I just have to run faster than you.'

But I suppose it means there'll be a witness.

The other thing frustrating thing about this particular call is that Mandy goes out. A lot, according to reports. She gets drunk, then spends her time wandering the corridors of the block shouting and causing trouble. There's an on-going spat with an ex-boyfriend who has recently moved in with another woman on the fourteenth. And any number of substance abusers scattered through the block mixing things up – socially as well as chemically. All in all, it sounds like a recipe for chaos, and not something that's going to lend itself to regular, well-apportioned community care. At a time of severe underfunding, it seems crazy to throw resources at a patient who has the capacity to decide whether they drink or eat or take drugs or not. It's a lifestyle choice – however severe that choice works itself out in practice.

But our community health team doesn't have the latitude or leverage to protest. The referrals come in, we go out.

The brief is to establish regular contact with Mandy. To get carers going in every day to encourage her to eat and get her used to some regularity in her life.

'It's only until a more regular provider can pick up' says the co-ordinator.

'I'm sorry I wasn't in earlier,' say Mandy. 'I had to go to the doctor's.'

'Oh? How did you get there?'

'Taxi,' she says. 'Well they're not going to come here, are they?'

'Ah'm on ma owen, as yoo ken no dowet see fer yerseln. Ma gel-fren, she's garn ta see them there Lady Boyz. So there ye hav'it. S'it. End of. A sorry tale, en'no mistakun. But ah'm very happy fer any'in yous tous can do ta help, y'kno wha ah mean? Ah'm ver' grateful.'

Rufus speaks so slowly it's like he's thumbing each word out in plasticine. Not only is he drunk but he has a strong Glaswegian accent, so it's almost impossible to understand what he's saying. The only way I can manage it is to completely relax, watch his mouth, and try to take clues from his inflections and sudden, wildly uncoordinated gestures. He's naked on the bed, which would be worrying if he wasn't so completely unbothered by it – in fact, much less self-conscious in his nudity than I am in my uniform. I can't help thinking about Rufus' girlfriend, sitting in the audience watching the immaculately made-up Lady Boys, their choreographed gestures, perfect diction, and wonder what she makes of the contrast.

Rufus smiles, exposing a mouth of greying stumps.

'[Translation] I suppose you've come to dress my wound? I'm sorry for the state I'm in, but I've had a few drinks and I lost track of where I was. I'm an alcoholic, you know. I'm cutting right down. I only had four cans. The doctor knows all about it. I've been on detox three times but nothing worked. That's just the way it is. Sometimes you just have to accept how things are I suppose. Do you know what I mean? Anyway – what about you? How are you? Thanks for coming. I really do appreciate everything you do.'

I've come with Jasmine, one of the Filipino nurses. To be honest, she's almost as hard to understand as Rufus. She speaks lightly and quickly, barely moving her mouth, strange intonations, swallowing some vowels, stopping unexpectedly on others, and ending every other sentence with an isn't it or a long, drawn-out aaaaah. Her small stature and delicate features completely belie her tough approach, though. She's small and busy and she's used to working fast. She tears open dressings kits, snaps gloves on and off, probes, irrigates, photographs, packs, re-dresses – all with a positivity that overwhelms any resistance. It's not that she's cold or harsh. Far from it. She has a kind of tough, Catholic love for everyone, including Rufus. Despite the alcohol I think he can feel it, too.

'I'm nah hurting you, am I?' she says, roughly prodding Aquacel into the wound.

'[Translation] No. You're alright. You carry on. I'm used to it. You're doing a fine job.'

'You know, you gah to take better care of yourself isn't it? It very durty down here, too much durty... How you ever going tah geh better? You listen tah me now. You geh wash now. I hep you.'

'[Translation] No. You're alright. Thanks for the offer but I'll just put on some clean underpants and have a wash later. It's no bother. You did a grand job. Thanks.'

I hand him some clean-ish Minion boxer shorts from a heap of clothing on the floor. By the time Rufus and I have figured out which way round they should go, Jasmine has packed her stuff away, disposed of the rubbish bag and started writing up her notes. She pauses to watch us, sighing heavily through her nose.

To be honest, anyone would sigh watching Rufus get his boxers on. He rolls around on the bed, waggling his long legs in the air, trying to put both through one hole, then taking them out and trying to put them both through the other hole, the whole time displaying with alarming clarity that which normally should not be displayed.

After a minute or two of this Jasmine sighs again, throws down her notes and intervenes.

'Give me dat,' she says. She slaps his legs down, rolls him onto his side, guides his left leg, then his right leg, says 'You bridge now...', and as soon as he does, she whips the boxers up with a satisfying snap of elastic.

'All done!' she says, winking at him. 'You guh boy.'

᪥

Strictly speaking, Mr Jeffries is a double-up.

Not for the usual reasons – manual handling issues, a history of aggressive behaviour, substance abuse, hazardous environment or a tendency to make accusations – but for something else, something unspecified. So far, I've been unable to get to the bottom of it, just a series of knowing smiles and nods. I'm supposed to visit Mr Jeffries to take blood, but unfortunately the nurse I was scheduled to go with has had to run out to a blocked catheter, and for one reason or another, there's no-one else.

'It's okay. I don't mind,' I tell Anna, the co-ordinator. 'I'm fine going on my own,'

'Are you sure, darlink? I'm so sorry there isn't anyone to go with you. But I'm sure you'll be fine. You used to work on ambulance before. I'm sure you've come across things a lot more – how should I say – strange.'

'In what way strange, exactly?'

'Just – you know – strange. Odd. Something different. But there's no danger involved and you are strong person so I'm sure you'll be fine. Just go in, get the blood and come out again.'

She smiles at me. 'Maybe like this...'

She frowns, crossing her arms across her chest.

'Why? Is it filthy in there?'

'No! Is not filthy. Is very nice.'

'What then? Is he a bit lecherous?'

'Lecherous? What is this lecherous?'

'You know. Hands everywhere.'

'No, darlink. No. He is not lecherous. You're perfectly safe as far as lecherous is concerned.'

'So what then?'

'You'll see. I'm perfectly happy for you to wait until someone becomes available…'

'It's fine. I'll go get the blood.'

'You are good boy. Very erm… how you say…?'

'I don't know. Brave?'

'No-ooo….'

'Foolhardy?'

She doesn't say what she means.

Mr Jeffries doesn't answer his phone, which is something the notes say is typical for him. He has a keysafe, though. The only thing is to go there and take a chance he's in.

Mr Jeffries lives on the top floor of a run-down block of flats. The architect must have designed the place in a rush over breakfast, because it's exactly like an upturned cereal box, with a lift at either end serving long, unbroken corridors of doors and security grilles. If by the day the block is austere, at night it's perfectly bleak. The lamp out front flickers, animating the entrance in such a menacing way I can't help zipping my jacket to the neck and shouldering my bag more squarely. Inside is worse, utterly lightless, with that heavy kind of dark you'd think was pumped in from deep underground. The corridor lights only come on when you move, and even then there's a delay, so the effect is of a steady falling forwards, disconcerting, not at all pleasant.

I knock on Mr Jeffries' door. There's a muffled answer. I use the key and let myself in.

The flat is warm, close, unaired, filled wall to ceiling with shelves and shelves of books – art, astrology, folklore, history, that kind of thing. Mr Jeffries is sitting in his lounge on an electric wheelchair, as perfectly contained in the glow from his desk lamp as a hunched insect preserved in amber.

He spins round to face me, and the first thing that strikes me are his eyes, wide-set and unblinking, tub-water grey, with a diverging bulge that gives him an acute and predatory appearance. That, coupled with his dry smile and knowing demeanour are as unsettling as you could get, and I suddenly understand why Anna thinks this is a double-up.

'I suppose you've come for my blood,' he says, arching his long fingers together and scrutinising me over the top of them. 'The doctor doesn't think I need it, but I think I know more about my condition than a simple GP. If only I had more energy – and a better prognosis – I'd sue them for millions. But really – what good would that do me?'

'I don't know,' I say.

'No. I don't suppose you do.'

He parts his hands in a simple gesture of letting go, but then his attitude hardens just as suddenly.

'Here's what I need you to do…' he says, and then tells me where to set up my things, what bottles to use, what the tests need to show and so on.

'Some people find me intimidating,' he says. 'My last consultant actually started to shake.'

'I don't think I'll shake,' I tell him, although it'll be a miracle if I don't. 'I'll save the shaking for afterwards.'

It helps when I find out that Mr Jeffries used to dialyse in the renal department around the time I was a ward clerk there. I don't remember him – and I feel sure I would – but it means we have a shared history of names and places I can use to distract him from focusing too much on me.

'No,' he says, interrupting a story about one of the PD nurses with red hair out of a bottle, 'not that vein. Use that one, there…'

It's annoying, but he's right. The blood starts to flow, and I'm immediately more relaxed.

'So, you had a transplant?' I say.

'I'll tell you a little story about that,' he says. 'The department had been having a run of deaths. A whole year of them. So much so that everyone was beginning to lose faith in their abilities. It was nothing to do with that, of course. But people divine all manner of things from simple coincidence. When it came to me, the consultant brought the kidney back himself, in a box on the backseat of his car. Can you imagine? It was a few years ago, of course. Things are different now.

Anyway, I was prepped and readied. Everyone wished me luck. And that was that. The next thing I knew, I was waking up in the recovery room. I was conscious of someone standing by the bed, and I thought it was a nurse. But when I turned to look, I saw a young woman, right beside me, staring down at me, with the oddest expression. Not sad – no. Not angry. Just – I don't know – confused. She stood there for the longest while. So long I couldn't bear it. I said Thank you for the kidney, closed my eyes, and prayed she would leave me alone. When I opened my eyes again the surgical team were standing around me, everyone smiling, waving blood results in the air, relieved the operation had been a success and their run of bad luck ended. Who was the girl who gave me the kidney? I asked them. She came to me. They dismissed my experience as post-operative hallucinations, and, of course, it was policy for them never to disclose any information about the donor. I knew it wasn't a hallucination, though. I've always been able to see things. Some people can. A little while later, just before I left the unit for good, I saw the consultant again. 'Who was she?' I asked him. 'Let's just say she was a woman who was formerly wealthy.' What does that mean – formerly wealthy? What do you think it means?'

'I don't know. It's an odd expression. Maybe he was speaking metaphorically. Maybe he meant wealth as in life, and formerly because she lost it.'

I tape some gauze to the crook of his arm. He gently holds his fingers to it, as if he's healing the wound by the power of touch.

'I never saw her again,' he says. 'Which is a shame, because she seemed so lost.'

And he turns his enormous eyes up to me, and I have to look away, because I don't want to see my own reflection contained in them.

'All done!' I say, shaking the vials of blood.

'Thank you,' he says. 'You've been most kind.'

'You're welcome.'

And he watches me closely as I pick up my things and go.

We've been told to double-up for this one, so Magda is sitting in her car outside the hostel, waiting.

'S'up!' she says, winding down the window.

'Any sign?'

'Nope.'

'They said he left the ward by taxi an hour ago.'

Magda shrugs and puts her phone in her pocket.

'Well I don't know what route crazy taxi driver took because no-one's been in or out since I've been here,' she says. 'and I've been here my whole life now. A proper stakeout. Wha'd'you suppose is in that pan?'

She nods and I turn to look: an orange saucepan on a window ledge outside the building.

'Dunno. Maybe it caught fire. Why? You can't be hungry.'

'Hungry, Jimmy? I've been gnawing the steering wheel.'

'That's the Christmas effect. Stretches everything.'

'Tell me about it. I've been googling the gastric band.'

I yawn, look up and down the street.

'Maybe he got dropped off just before you came, Magda.'

'All right. I suppose we should knock, then.'

She squeezes out of the car, hauls her bags from the boot, and we both go up the stoop to the front door. There's a carrier bag of empty jam jars on the top step with a note tied to the top.

For Janice.

Magda pushes the button marked Manager on the intercom. There's a long dialling tone, followed by a crackly voice from some remote location.

Scheme manager mouths Magda, then leans into the intercom.

'Hello. It's nurses from hospital. Come to see Frankie.'

The voice says something we can't understand. A pause, then the door buzzes and I shoulder it open. There's another, inner security door – and just as I realise that we need to be buzzed through that, too, the intercom rings off.

Magda frowns.

'You're gonna have to be quicker than that, Jimmy boy' she says, then goes back out onto the stoop to push the button again. Another wait. The intercom crackles again, but this time the inner door clicks without any words being said.

'You've done this before,' says Magda.

'What?' says the voice.

'I said we're in now, thanks very much.'

The lobby has the beaten, low-lit and musty atmosphere of hostels the world over. Some of the doors have numbers, some of them just the ghosts of numbers. Many of them have been kicked-in and repaired, painted and repainted so many times the panels and joints of the wood have a gloopy, approximate look.

Magda knocks on Frankie's door. There's no reply.

'Did you ring his mobile?'

'It went to voicemail.'

'Try again.'

We both hear it ringing from inside the room.

'So he's either ignoring us, gone out again and left his phone, or he's lying on the floor. Either way we're going to have to do something.'

'Let's see if scheme manager has a key.'

Magda goes back to the intercom to explain the situation; I put a bag down to stop the inner door closing again, then go back to the steps beside Frankie's room and knock a few more times, putting my ear to the door to see if I can hear anyone moving.

'He'll be over in five minutes,' says Magda, coming back. 'Anything?'

'Nah. I don't think he's in.'

We wait for the scheme manager.

There's a door marked Private just behind Magda.

'What d'you think's through there?'

'I don't know, Jimmy. Wonderland, probably.'

Magda checks her phone again.

'What are you looking up now?'

'Places to eat.'

Even though he sounded miles away on the intercom, the scheme manager is with us in five minutes. Graham completely fills the hallway, so tall and powerfully built I wouldn't be surprised to hear that his DNA was ten percent Viking, fifteen oak.

'He'll be in the hospital,' he says, pulling an enormous fob of keys from his parka pocket and squeezing between us to the door.

'But he's only just come out!'

Graham looks at me and smiles.

'I'm guessing you haven't met Frankie before?'

'No.'

Graham presses his lips and shakes his head.

'It's always the same. They say medically ready for discharge, Frankie hears it as medically ready for drinking. He'll have got the taxi driver to drop him at the nearest off-licence.'

Graham knocks on the door, calls out, then puts one of his keys in the lock and lets us in.

'See?' he says. 'Empty.'

A scattering of filthy clothes, food cartons, random stuff. The bed is rucked up, seamy – bloody, even, especially the pillows.

'He fell over and whacked his head,' says Graham. 'That's why he went in this last time.'

Frankie's phone is on the table. Graham picks it up and balances it in his hand like an urban tracker able to tell where the owner was, what they were thinking, where they were heading, simply by the weight.

'He must've come by to pick up some money and left his phone,' he says, then carefully puts it down again.

'We'll follow it up, reschedule then let you know,' says Magda.

'Thanks,' says Graham. 'You know – Frankie's the sweetest guy. Everyone's done their best, but it's hopeless, really. He had everything. Great job. Pillar of the community. But something happened somewhere along the line and he drifted off track. Who knows? Whatever it was it's turned him into the world's slowest suicide. Anyway! There you are! Thanks for dropping by! And a Happy New

Year...!'

He shows us out and waves when we turn to look.

At the bottom of the stoop we pause to let a young family go by: a bearded guy in a red check shirt and Timberland boots, having an earnest discussion on the phone whilst he pushes a baby in a pram, and a tiny boy carefully skips along the pavement beside him.

'What do you think?' says Magda as we watch them go. 'Maybe that is Frankie's problem. Maybe he stepped on a crack when he was little.'

'Mexican liqueur. Seven letters. Beginning with T.'

'Tequila?'

'Is that a liqueur?'

'It's made from a cactus. Does that count? Anyway, I can't think of any other specifically Mexican drinks. Apart from Dos Equis.'

'What on earth is Dos Equis?'

'A beer. I think.'

'Well. Let's go with tequila then, shall we? And see how we get on...'

Marilyn had a fall in the early hours and tore her arm. She's busy filling in the crossword whilst I'm delicately cleaning the wound, soaking it in saline, gently replacing the skin flap as best I can, then patting the area dry ready for the steri-strips. Her version of events was that she stumbled over some shoeboxes – no mention of the copious amounts of whisky she'd put away in the hours leading up. If she sees the irony in our conversation about booze, she doesn't show it.

'Oh I'm terribly sorry. I misread the clue,' she says. 'It actually says Mexican liquor. These glasses are absolutely no good at all.'

'Definitely tequila then.'

'...which makes one down agora. Which fits! Well done!'

Marilyn is a high-functioning alcoholic. She has a beautiful house in the centre of town, filled with paintings and books, sculptures and

133

peculiar antiques, everything brilliantly lit by the sunshine that positively bounds in through the open patio doors.

'You have a lovely house,' I tell her, applying the first layer of dressing.

'That's sweet of you,' she says.

'How long have you lived here?'

'Too long. But you know, when Teddy and I moved here in the seventies, it was a different street altogether. Everyone knew each other. It was all terribly friendly and interesting. But now it's simply overrun with cars, no-one has any time for anything, and the only contact you have is with the postman. Speaking of which…'

Keeping her bad arm as still as she can, she rummages around the clutter on the table and produces a Royal Mail missed delivery card.

'Look at that!' she says. 'Sorry we missed you! What on earth do they mean? Sorry we missed you! I've been in all blessed day! I simply fail to understand how they could have crept up the front steps and dropped that through the letterbox without me hearing a thing. Honestly, they must be employing cat burglars or something. Or maybe he ties rags round his shoes. It's enough to drive you absolutely insane!'

'You'd think he'd want to drop it off, though, just to lighten his bag.'

'Lighten his bag! I'll lighten his bag when I get hold of him.'

'Almost done,' I tell her.

'Smashing,' she says, lowering her glasses from the top of her head back down on to the tip of her nose, as she goes back to the crossword.

'Fifteen across. Famous Bohemian. Beginning with M.'

She snorts.

'Well – I'd be very tempted to write Marilyn – but unfortunately it ends in an A'.

7: Relativity

Mrs Butterworth is wearing a cornflower blue chenille dressing gown, its plump collar falling open at the neck. She talks in a soft, sadly undifferentiated way, like fog flowing over the brow of a hill. And whilst she talks, she gently rubs the side of her tummy, in the unconscious way pregnant women sometimes stroke their bumps, although the last time Mrs Butterworth was pregnant it was back in the sixties, and the swelling in her abdomen is now diverticula disease. Behind her on the wall is a photograph – the seventies, I'd guess – Mrs Butterworth in the centre, smiling brightly, her arms left and right around a smart looking boy standing straight-backed, and a younger girl with bright yellow hair, leaning forwards, her face a little out of shot.

'Gilly's not a bad daughter. She's got her own problems. It goes back a long way. It's all diagnosed. She's been on Prozac for twenty years or more. Who knows what she'd be like if she ever came off. She's had therapy and a few stays in hospital, but nothing seems to do the trick. She's just fundamentally unhappy, I suppose, and I can't help blaming myself. But it's just – I don't know – what with my recent scare and all this and that, I wish it could be different. Like normal families. My eldest child Peter, he lives in Australia, and he does what he can from there. He rings every other day and whenever his business takes him this way he makes a point of stopping over. What do you need? he'll say. Just like that. Name it. He's such a good boy. You wouldn't think they came from the same place. I know he gets cross with Gilly, but he holds it back because he knows it'll only make things worse. There's nothing anyone can do. It's such a shame. She only lives three streets away but I'll tell you something: Australia seems closer. I haven't seen her since January. To be fair, she did come to the hospital with me that time, when I went in for the operation. I mean – it was a serious thing. They didn't know if I'd come out of it. I had to sign papers. And the morning of the operation, there I was, sitting in bed waiting to get wheeled through, with this terrible thing hanging over me, and Gilly was pacing up and down, sighing like she does, checking her phone every five seconds. And then she turns round to me and she says I can't wait here all day. I've got things to do! And she left. And that was that. I didn't make a fuss. I knew it wouldn't help. I told Peter about it and I know he was furious, but what could he do? I think he did ring her, though, because when I was discharged she came over to see me. I kept the conversation as light as I could. I mean – what was there to say? But my grandson, James – not the most prepossessing boy in the world. Well James was sitting on this chair with his head down in his phone, jabbing away with his thumbs, and it was all very quiet, so I just thought I'd ask him about school. Right! That's it! she said. I don't have to stand here and listen to this! And they left. And that was the last I heard from them. Although I did try ringing her last week, when I needed a bulb changing in the living room. Her husband Trevor answered the phone. Well. He's not what you might call an attentive son-in-law. Do you know what he said to me? He said Can't you just stand on a ladder and do it? Me! On a ladder! That's okay, Trevor I said. I'm getting used to living in the dark.'

Melvin is as landed and unfortunate in his armchair as a hippo in the dry season. An affable hippo, though, in a taut, custard yellow, California Dreamin' t-shirt and grey jogging bottoms, his enormous hands restlessly picking at the padding of the arm rests, as if he's gauging the right moment to tear them off and throw them.

'What were you saying?' he says. 'I lost the thread.'

He laughs, exposing a few raw and stumpy teeth. If I had a head of cabbage, I'd chuck it, watch him crunch it down, waggle his ears.

'He does that a lot,' says Bibi, Melvin's wife. 'Lose the thread, I mean.'

If Melvin is the hippo in this relationship, Bibi is the little bird that rides on his head. A trim, quick figure, she's constantly up and down, repositioning cushions, fetching beakers of juice, a towel, a diary, a snack, another beaker of juice. She smiles at me and surreptitiously touches the side of her head, turning the gesture into an innocent scratch of her eyebrow when Melvin unexpectedly glances her way.

'So what's the plan, chief?' says Melvin. 'What're you going to do with me? Drag me off to the knackers yard, I 'spect. I'd make a lot of glue.'

'Don't say that!' says Bibi, jumping up again to move the stool so he can reposition his feet.

'Ahh!' he booms. 'Thanks Beebs.'

The situation has been a long time coming and it's hard to know where to start. Diabetes, joint damage, skin infections, kidney and liver issues – the list neatly packaged-up in the phrase comorbidities. Things were difficult enough before his latest fall, but he's been discharged from hospital with a bandaged foot and the results of an MRI confirming mixed dementia. There's a lot to think about.

'Today's a good day,' says Bibi. 'Isn't it darling?'

'Every day's a good day,' says Melvin.

'Well,' says Bibi. 'Mostly.'

She's doing her best to cope, but it's a struggle. She's already told me about his mood swings, how he'll be fine one minute and raging the next. There's a shine to her eyes that's so brittle I don't know if she's ready to sob, scream or laugh out loud.

'But where are my manners?' she says. 'Can I get you anything?'

'No, no! That's kind of you but I'm fine, thanks.'

'Just let me know. It's no trouble.'

Melvin is sitting in front of a large white blind. The blind has been pulled down to shield him from the midday sun. Now and again the shadow of a seagull glides across the blind, so clearly you can even see the toes of its webbed feet and the way it flicks its head from side to side. Down in the street some workmen have finished lunch. They're shouting and swearing, starting up the mixer, tapping off bricks for a new wall.

'Hear that?' says Melvin. 'I expect that's the seagull, building his nest.'

We all laugh.

He clasps his hands across his belly, waggles his ears.

∽

Carl climbs back into bed and slowly pulls the covers up to his chin. He's a frail, tentative man in his forties, skin like parchment paper, his teeth sharp and defined. I'm surprised he's been discharged home like this, but then again, he's a convincing witness, and they're short of beds on the psych wards.

'I'm over it,' he says. 'I won't be trying to kill myself again.' He grimaces, and pulls the covers even more tightly around him.

This last time was the second attempt. Carl had taken an overdose of medication he'd stored up over time. He'd panicked at the last minute and called a friend, who'd dialled 999. When the paramedics broke the door down Carl was in cardiac arrest. They managed to get him back, though, and after a prolonged stay in hospital – a couple of weeks in intensive care, a month on the wards – he'd been discharged home with community support.

It's a nice flat, but so bare you'd think Carl had just moved in. Even though he's an artist, there are no pictures on the walls apart from two, childish, brightly-coloured crayon drawings of a dragon and a butterfly. The bare boards seem to go on for miles, from Carl's bedroom at the back of the house to the huge bay windows at the front. By the bed he has an alarm clock and a glass of water. At the foot of the bed is a stuffed toy: Tigger, from Winnie the Pooh.

'Tigger saved my life,' says Carl. 'When I came out of ITU I only had the strength to stroke his head. It gave me power, though. Sounds silly but it's true. He was my best friend in there. He kept me going, stood up for me. I mean – ITU was the worst. It was a nightmare. You'd think I was unconscious to look at me, but I wasn't. Everything was out to get me – the equipment, the nurses. Everything was holding me down trying to climb inside me. I struggled like mad. One time I even threw myself out of bed. I just climbed over the cot sides and ended up on the floor – drips, lines, cables, the lot. Everyone came running. I thought they were coming to finish me off so I fought like crazy. Then they sent me back under. Next thing I knew Dad was standing by the bed on the ward. He looked so old and sad and worn out. It was Dad who gave me the spare kidney when I needed it, a few years ago. He's amazing, my Dad. He came all the way down from Scotland to see me. On the train. That's a long way! I just kept thinking about him, sitting there, staring out the window. But when he got here I didn't know what to say to him. Other than sorry, obviously. The worst thing was, when he left me at the hospital he came back here to sleep – in this bed, where I did the deed. That made me feel very strange. But he couldn't afford a hotel, so I suppose it made sense. I wondered how I'd cope, coming back to this flat. It's been alright, though. I don't think about it all that much. Funny, isn't it?'

Vera is as formidable as an oak tree. An ancient, wonderfully craggy version, a boundary oak, maybe, with a disposition of knots and old storm wounds that give her a ferocious but at the same time peculiarly forbearing and kindly expression.

'How did I get like this?' she says, approximating a walk by rocking from side to side in her vast, rose-pink slippers, pulling the cord of her dressing gown so tight I'm worried her curlers will fly off. 'Dear oh dear. Sad, innit?'

She stops and gives me a baleful look.

'Don't get old,' she says.

'What's the alternative?'

'What's the alternative? Switzerland.'

She shakes her head and carries on into the living room.

'Make yourself at home,' she says, waving dismissively at the sofa, then slowly lowering herself into a well-worn armchair. 'Mind you, I've lived here sixty year and I still 'ain't managed it.'

'I don't know. Seems like a nice place.'

'You make the best, d'oncha?' she says, putting her feet up with an expressive range of ooh-ooh-ooh's and aah's.

'All right?' I ask her. 'Do you need a hand?'

'I need more than a hand,' she says. 'What else've you got?'

Before I manage to do anything, the phone rings. Vera mutters a great deal as she picks up the phone from the side table, holding it to the end of her nose to scrutinise the number, then making a great fuss of holding it at arm's length to press the ok button, frowning at the same time, as if she was being asked to do something outrageous, then cautiously and slowly putting the phone to her ear. I can hear the voice on the other end shouting as the phone travels through the air – a man's voice, saying Nan, Nan, It's John. Nan?

'21364' she says, in a strangely formal voice. But that only lasts as long as it takes to establish it's John on the other end, and she immediately slumps back into normal Vera again. I prepare the paperwork and get my obs kit out, whilst Vera sighs and tuts and does her best to reassure John she's all right, and no, she's all right as far as shopping goes, she's got enough to last her till Christmas, and yes, she'll let him know how the appointment goes, and no, she doesn't want anyone to worry, she hasn't lived till ninety without learning a thing or two. There's a moment towards the end of the conversation when John seems to be telling her something about himself.

'Oh? …. What's that, then? …. You what?…. I thought that was cows..?'

She looks at me, raising her eyebrows and shaking her head, then refocuses her attention on what John has to say.

'Righto, then, John. You get better soon, love. And love to the kids. All right? All right? Bye bye, John. Bye bye.'

She thumbs the phone off with the same pantomime of attention as the answering of it, then drops it back with the TV guide on the side table.

'That was John,' she says.

'Oh?'

'Yes. He's always ringing me up to ask how I am and then telling me he's got it worse.'

'Why? What's the matter with him?'

'Foot and mouth, he says. I thought that was something cows got.'

'He probably means hand foot and mouth. It's a viral thing…'

'Oh. I see,' she says, but I can tell she doesn't. 'That's all right, then.'

She pats her curlers and rearranges her dressing gown whilst she gets her thoughts in order.

'Only John!' she says at last. 'He's a bloody postman! Although saying that, maybe they gave him a new round that takes in a farm somewhere.'

'Maybe,' I say.

She sighs and shakes her head.

'Hark at me!' she says. 'I've turned into a right old miserable moo!'

There's a three-quarter length, black and white portrait of Madeleine on the shelf behind her: a young woman in her early twenties, I'd guess, in a French beret and raincoat, sitting in the driving seat of an open-topped sports car. She's resting her left elbow on the door, right hand on the steering wheel, staring at the camera in a wry and open-faced way, as if she knows – and the photographer knows – that any moment now she'll be tearing off that beret, throwing it aside and racing off down the road in a scattering of gravel.

Seventy years have past, and much has changed, but Madeleine is looking at me with exactly the same expression.

'I suppose you've come to jab me again,' she says.

'I'm afraid so.'

'Let's get on with it, then.'

She watches me whilst I fill in the Tinzaparin chart and check the syringe.

'Married?' she says.

'I am, yes. Eighteen years.'

'Marvellous,' she says. 'I was married twice, you know.'

'Really?'

'Both times for exactly thirty years. To the day.'

'That's – consistent.'

'My first husband was alright, I suppose, but I think essentially we just didn't mesh.'

'Thirty years. That's a long time not to mesh.'

'One put up with these things. Unlike today, of course. Today it's like cancelling the papers. George was terribly romantic to begin with, but that petered out and in the end we were more like brother and sister. Until he went bankrupt, and started to drink an awful lot more, and then life became rather sticky.'

'In what way?'

'He became bitter about everything. The fact we never had children. The constant moving about. He didn't like what I had, you see, which is a very strong sense of self. I think he was really rather threatened by that, and I'm afraid he became something of a bully. He hit me, you know.'

'I'm sorry to hear that.'

'The first time I said to him George. You do that once more and I'll be off. And although he did make an effort to change his ways for a week or two, the writing was on the wall in jolly big letters. He hit me again. Hard, across the face. So hard in fact that I fell backwards into a rose bush. Scratched my stockings and my legs. I was in a frightful state. Anyway, I picked myself up with as much dignity as I could muster, walked myself back into the house, packed a suitcase, and I left him, and I never went back. And there! That was the first thirty years.'

'So then what happened?'

'I thought that was that, of course. I was off men for good. But actually what I was off was marriage. And I started to have quite a nice time of it. No responsibilities. I like to think of that time as my golden period. Then I met Pierre. Lovely, sad Pierre. French, y'know. From Paris. I told him I didn't want anything serious, but he kept on and on

142

in that terribly sad and attractive way he had, and eventually I said Look. We can live together if you like. But that's as far as I'm prepared to go. So that's what we did. We lived together for a year or so, and then I thought, well – what the hell? Why not? And we were married, and everything changed again. You see I'd been worried I'd end up with someone like my first husband. What I wanted was someone who was so unlike me there wouldn't be any clashes. And Pierre and I were certainly different. He was from a terribly poor background, you see. During the war he'd lived out in the mountains, with the resistance. They didn't even have any shoes, and had to tie newspaper round their feet, creeping into the valley at night to scavenge whatever they could, and lay traps for the Germans. He was captured, I'm afraid, and ended up in a concentration camp. And that was a frightful business. I'm certain it was the source of all his sadness.'

'It's hard to imagine how awful it must have been for him.'

'Pierre didn't ever talk to me about it, though, and I think in the end that was the problem. One day he came home, and instead of walking through to give me a kiss, he went into the bathroom and locked the door. Well I knew straightaway something was wrong, because we didn't ever lock the door if it was just the two of us. So after a while I went to the bathroom and knocked. He wouldn't answer, but I kept on and in the end he told me to go away. I did – for as long as I could bear. Then I went back to the bathroom and I knocked again. Pierre? I said. What on earth's the matter? And he didn't answer, and he didn't answer... so I just kept knocking, and I said if he didn't let me in I'd break the door down. Which sounds pretty hot stuff but it was only a token kind of lock. So that's what I did. I pushed the door in, and there he was, sitting on the toilet, his head resting against the wall, looking into space. You're scaring me I said. What's wrong? But he couldn't or wouldn't say, so I called the ambulance. They took him away, and he died three days later.'

'That's awful! Do you know what the problem was?'

Madeleine slowly gathers her blouse an inch so I can inject her in the abdomen.

'They were never terribly specific and I was too upset to inquire. Men's trouble, something of that nature,' she says, flinching as the needle goes in. 'So there we are. That was the end of it. Thirty years to the day. And now here I am, an old woman being jabbed in the tummy, wondering what on earth all the fuss was about.'

She lowers her blouse and settles herself in the chair again.

'But there are always compensations,' she says.

'I suppose,' I say, posting the used syringe into the sharps bin and peeling off my blue gloves. 'That's a very balanced way of looking at it. What sort of compensations?'

'Well – in my case, a simply marvellous view of the sea!'

Stepping through the front door into Mary's house is like stepping into a crazy echo chamber. There's a radio playing full blast in the kitchen, a TV in the front room with loud music and studio applause, and a TV in the back room with explosions and machine gun fire. The whole effect is made worse by the fact that the house has laminate flooring, and there's not much in the way of soft furnishings. When I call Mary's name to announce myself I have to shout. Her four-wheeled walker is at a strange angle in the middle of the hall, like she dumped it there in a hurry. I'm worried something's happened, but as soon as I go forward to put it straight, she emerges from a tiny bathroom under the stairs.

'I said go through,' she says. 'Didn't you hear me?'

'Well it's quite noisy, Mary. D'you mind if I turn things down a bit?'

'Suit yourself,' she says, then takes the walker from me and walks with it through into the back room, her shoulders hunched, rolling heavily in the hip, like an old farmer ploughing a muddy field.

I do a quick tour of the house, switching off the TV and the radio. It only leaves the TV in the back room, a giant plasma affair. It's playing a forties war film. There's a close-up of John Mills looking tense, which feels about right as I ask Mary if she'd mind turning it off

144

for a bit.

'You do it,' she says.

I can't see the remote, so I just touch what looks like the off button on the bottom of the screen. The whole thing immediately dumps to a white fuzz accompanied by a hideous noise.

'Oh what've you done now?' she says, producing the remote from her cardigan pocket and zapping it off. 'Good God almighty!'

'There! That's better!' I say. 'I couldn't hear myself think.'

She raises her eyebrows, like she could say a few things about that if she wanted to.

'How are you feeling?' I ask her.

'Much the same,' she says. 'Terrible.'

'I'm sorry to hear that. In what way terrible?'

'What?'

'I say in what way terrible?'

'What d'you mean?'

'Are you in pain?'

'No. Thank God.'

'Do you feel sick? Dizzy? Short of breath?'

'No.'

'Lacking in energy?'

'I do my best.'

'I'm sure you do. So when you say you feel terrible, what... erm....'

She's ignoring me now, fussing with a heap of stuff next to her on the sofa, so I decide not to push the "feeling terrible" thing any further and see if her obs offer any clues instead.

'Would you mind if I did your blood pressure and temperature and so on?' I ask her, unzipping my bag.

'Be my guest,' she says, and immediately rolls up the sleeve of her cardigan.

Just behind her on the wall is a large, three part picture frame, a photo of the Queen on the left looking a little dazed, a royal letter on the right, and the two panels separated by a golden tassel like a light pull or a curtain closer. I wonder what would happen if the glass wasn't there and you could reach in and pull it. Maybe the national anthem would play and then the whole thing would burst into flames.

'What's that for?' I ask her.

'We were married sixty years,' she says.

'Wow! That's lovely.'

'He's gone now.'

'I'm sorry.'

'What can you expect?'

'I suppose.'

'He built this place.'

'Did he? That's amazing.'

'He was a builder.'

'Yes. I bet he must've worked hard.'

'He never stopped.'

'Sixty years! That's very impressive, Mary. You'll have to tell me your secret.'

'What secret?'

'How you managed to stay married for sixty years.'

'I couldn't think what else to do. Besides, you get used to someone.'

'I suppose that's true. So how did you two meet?'

'He tripped me up in Woolworth's.'

'Where? By the pick n'mix?'

'All I know is, his friend was going with my friend.'

She sighs and looks pained, as if the effort of remembering these things is exhausting her.

'That didn't last,' she says. 'Are you done now or what?'

It's already late when I get there, the sun low on the hills, shreds of pink cloud against a deepening sky.

Roy answers the door with a tea cloth in his hands.

'Come on in!' he says, flipping the cloth over his shoulder, shaking my hand warmly and ushering me in. 'Jean's just through here. She will be pleased to see you.'

He follows me into the living room, dragging his left foot a little, like his hips are starting to go.

'What a pair we are!' he says. 'A job lot. Aren't we Jean? A job lot?'

Jean is sitting by the patio window in a high-backed armchair, smiling at us both with as much of a delighted expression as her stroke will allow. She tries to speak, too, and though it's incomprehensible, Roy seems to know what she means, and fills in the gaps.

I've come to change the dressing on her arm. For some reason she can't help picking and scratching at it, and the wounds have become infected.

'I did clip the nails on her hand,' says Roy, 'but she was still finding a way through it all. Weren't you, Jean?'

He strokes her hair. 'Thanks again for coming out. We do appreciate it.'

'It's no trouble.'

He stands over me whilst I prepare the dressings.

'I have to apologise if I smell a little – you know.'

'I can't smell anything,' I tell him. 'Why – what have you had? Garlic sausage?'

'Me? No! A little glass of whisky.'

'I think you're more than entitled to a glass of whisky. What sort is it?'

'Famous Grouse.'

'That's a good one,' I say, sounding as if I know about these things. To back it up, I tell him about a job I used to have a few years ago, working for a company that maintained intranets. 'One of the clients ran a gin distillery,' I tell him. 'They showed us round once. It was amazing! These gigantic stills, filling the place, right up to the roof, like giant copper onions.'

Roy laughs.

'I wouldn't mind seeing that,' he says. 'Mind you – I'm not really a gin man.'

I start cutting off the old bandage. Jean watches me with her eyes wide and her mouth hanging open.

'Alright?' I say. 'I'm just going to use a little bit of sterile water...'

Roy helps out where he can, passing me things, comforting Jean, keeping her distracted. It's all pretty straightforward and I'm done in a few minutes.

'There! Good as new!' I say, peeling off my gloves and starting to clear up.

'Here! You might be interested to see this..' says Roy. He unhooks a framed, black and white picture from the wall. A man in overalls, neckerchief and peaked cap standing on the tracks beside an enormous steam engine.

'I used to work the locomotives. A fireman to begin with, until I made driver. It's funny to think of it now, y'know, but on an early turn I used to stop off on the way into the yard for a pint of Guinness. Not for the alcohol, y'understand. For the oomph. I tell you what – it was hard work, shovelling coal, keeping it going. But it was the best job in the world. You got into a sort of flow after a while, and there was nothing you couldn't do. I'd be all the way to Newcastle and back, and I'd suddenly think hang on a minute! I haven't had a wee since breakfast! But that's how it was.'

We both look at the picture for a moment. Roy has one hand on the rail of the cab, one foot on the plate, and he's standing looking at the camera with such a strong and confident gaze you'd think for tuppence he could pick the whole thing up and wave it over his head.

'These days the only exercise I get is wheeling Jean along the front,' he says, wiping the glass with his elbow and then carefully hanging it back on the wall. 'But we do alright, don't we Jean? Hey?'

He bends down to give her a kiss on the cheek, and she gives him a big, adoring smile in return, before turning her attention to the new bandage, looking for any weak spots with her other hand.

Melvin answers the door in his pants. He's quite a sight. Wild white hair sweeping back from his head, a long, ginger-white goatee to match; perfectly round grey-blue eyes, and the kind of ravaged and rangy body you might see trotting alongside your jeep on the Serengeti.

He doesn't speak. He just stands there, staring at me, one hand on the door, one hand adjusting himself.

'Hello!' I say. 'My name's Jim. From the Rapid Response Team. I've come to see Helen.'

He smiles suddenly, a wide, gummy affair, but makes no other sign that he's understood what I've just said.

'Here's my badge,' I say, holding it up.

He glances at it, then carries on staring at me.

'Is it okay if I come in and see her, d'you think? Helen?' I pause. 'Is she in?'

He opens the door wider, still holding on to it, which I take as an invitation to come in. It's a squeeze to get past him, though, especially with all my bags. The hallway is so tiny there's barely room for the two of us. I'm expecting Melvin to make some room, but he doesn't.

'I'll take my shoes off,' I say, struggling in the cramped space. 'It's a bit wet outside.'

'If you don't mind,' he says, suddenly animated, as if the last minute or so was just a technical glitch. 'We've had so many people in and out.'

'No worries,' I say. 'I bought these shoes 'cos they're easy to slip on and off. There! Good! Okay! So – shall we go through...?'

The sitting room is swelteringly hot. The gas fire's on all-bars, and the air ripples above a free-standing radiator (all of which explains the pants). Melvin hops over to his chair and goes through an athletic, sitting down routine, involving him taking his weight on his arms, raising his legs, lowering himself slowly, then folding his bony arms and legs and smiling with a self-satisfied leer.

Helen waves me over.

'Ignore him,' she says.

The examination is straightforward. Everything's fine. Helen's recovering well and she's happy to be home. I tell her we'll be discharging her from our service, but that it's easy for us to come back if anything changes.

Melvin watches the whole procedure with intense interest. Whilst I'm writing up the notes, he starts talking again.

'I played a lot of football,' he says, as if I'd asked. 'A lot of football. But it did my head in. Have you heard that before?'

'D'you mean sport and head injuries? I think I heard something.'

'It's the big leather balls. Laces down the middle. I played centre forward. I was heading it all the time.'

'I suppose it wouldn't do your brain much good. All that shaking. Like boxers.'

'I did boxing, too. And rugby. You bang your head a lot in rugby.'

'You certainly do.'

'But football was the main thing. I did all the trials. I played semi-professionally for years. One game I scored eleven goals. This guy comes up to me after, and he says How'd you do it, Melvin? How'd you score all them goals? And I says to him What goals? I don't know what you mean, mate. The ball comes to me, something happens, it's in the net. That's it. It's a natural thing, like breathing. They sent me to Germany.'

'Did they?'

'This German coach, he runs over to me. He leans in ... like this ... and he wags his finger in my face... like this ... and he says You! You're the man with all the goals. You're a professional. You shouldn't be here. So I says to him Mate! What goals? I don't know what you're talking about. The ball comes over – it's on my head – it's in the net. That's it. It's got nothing to do with me.'

'How'd he take it?'

'How'd who take what?'

'The German manager. How'd he take hearing about all the goals?'
Melvin shrugs.

'He could see,' he says. 'He knew what he had there.'

'So then what happened?'

'I came back, didn't I? Got a job in a laundry. And here we all are!'

'Just ignore him,' says Helen.

∽

Moira's mouth has a tragic and graven quality, down-turned, thinly incised, which, along with her hooded eyelids and watery blue eyes, gives her a profoundly disapproving expression, something you could imagine at Judgement Day, looking out across the smoking ruins of the world, with a caption in Gothic script that read: I told you so.

'I spent a great deal on his education so it's about time he started paying some of it back,' she says, the point of her elbow dug into the armrest so she can hold her bandaged hand straight up in the air like a courtroom exhibit.

'When did you last see him?'

'Simon? Yesterday. He stayed the absolute minimum and then he was off to another meeting. I said to him: What's more important – work, or the health of your mother? I won't be here much longer. If it's going to go on like this, the sooner I go, the better.'

'Where does Simon live?'

'Where doesn't he live. It's absurd. He's got enormous houses all over the place and he spends most of his time in hotels.'

'Couldn't you move in with him?'

She turns her eyes on me.

'He's a businessman, dear. Not a saint.'

It's been a long and difficult assessment. Moira has the issue of her hand, of course, but it strikes me that her biggest problem is depression, a bleak and palpable thing that sucks all the light and life from the air, like a black hole opened up in a riser-recliner and someone tried to disguise it with a dressing-gown.

'I asked Jenny upstairs if she could go out and get me a paper. And d'you know what she said?'

'What did she say?'

'She said No.'

'No?'

'No. Just like that.'

'Pretty harsh.'

'Harsh? I've known her twenty years. I think it's positively murderous.'

She pats her hair with her bad hand and then winces as she lowers it back to her lap.

'I shan't be bothering her again,' she says.

The phone rings. Moira mutters and frowns.

'Shall I get it for you?' I say.

'I'm not dead yet,' she says, and then makes a huge, sighing deal of picking up, reciting the name of the town and the phone number when the handset eventually makes it up to her ear, as brave as a telephonist being martyred at the stake, making one last connection amongst the flames.

Oh. It's you... Well how d'you think I'm getting on? ... I'm not, and that's the whole point... Yes, he's here now... How should I know what he thinks? He just sits there making approximate noises... Not at the moment, no. I haven't finished with him yet. When I have I'll get him to call you... Yes, thank you. I think I have everything I need – excepting a son who gives a damn.

And she hangs up.

'That was Simon.'

'I guessed.'

She observes me closely.

'He sends his regards,' she says, after a very long while.

Parkinson's disease has robbed Terry of facial expression, but from his sparkling eyes I can tell he's very keen to tell me how he met his wife. Her pictures are everywhere in the flat, a studio portrait of a young woman leaning forwards in a serious, three-quarter pose; shots of her in a wedding dress; cuddling babies; making a speech; holding a hat on her head on the deck of a boat – all with a kind of Doris Day glow, and vastly outnumbering the various other family photos dotted about the place.

'She died ten years ago,' he says. 'I just want to be with her now. Not in a creepy way. It's just how it is.'

'I can understand that.'

'Do you want to know how we met? It's a funny story. Have you time?'

I tell him I definitely want to hear it, but can he sit down first. 'Because honestly, Terry – if I hadn't been standing here with my wicket keeper's mitts on, you would've pitched head first into the bookcase. I can fetch whatever you need. Come on! Let me help you to a chair.'

'Just a sec,now – just a sec,' he says, turning stiffly on the spot and almost plunging backwards into a pile of records.

'Whoa! Look – why not have a seat here? I'll make you a drink and then we can talk about what to do next. And you can tell me how you met your wife.'

He seems to accept this, but instead of heading for the nearest sofa, leads me across the cluttered flat to a dangerously low Ottoman.

'This'll do,' he says, shuffling carefully into position, and then, whilst he's still miles away, unexpectedly launching himself backwards stiff as a puppet whose strings have been snatched up to throw it back in the trunk. He catches me off guard. I grab the front of his shirt to stop him whacking his head on the wall. The shirt makes an impressive ripping noise.

'Sorry Terry!'

'Don't worry! Don't worry!' he says. 'It's a cheap old thing. I've got hundreds. I'll just go fetch another...'

He starts trying to get up again. It's a job to stop him.

What with one thing and another, Terry needs to go to hospital. Whilst we sit together waiting for the ambulance, he finally gets round to telling me the anecdote about his wife.

'You wouldn't think to look at me now, but back then I wasn't entirely hopeless. I was studying architecture at university. A good friend of mine was doing medicine. C'mon Terry! he said. There's a party at the local hospital. All the hot nurses will be there. Well I couldn't say no to that, could I? Turns out it was a big old psychiatric hospital in the suburbs, which put me off a bit, but – well – hot nurses and all that. So we sneaked inside, and there was a long, long corridor, the kind of corridor you see in your dreams, that goes on forever. And coming down this corridor, floating towards us out of the light, were two of the most gorgeous nurses you'd ever seen in your life. One a redhead, the other blond. And we were both so dumbstruck we couldn't do or say anything, we just sort of stepped helplessly to the side. Except there was fresh wax on the floor under the radiator, and I was wearing my shoes with the shiny soles. So I went flying arse over apex and ended up kicking the blond one in the rear. Two years later we were married. So whenever anyone asks me, How did you meet your wife? I tell them I was in a psychiatric hospital and I kicked one of the nurses.'

8: Time, Place and Other Confusions

Maud's designated next of kin, Alan, lets me in. A tidy man in his early sixties, his grey beard is as scrupulously clipped and pressed as his Nordic woolly jumper.

'Just through there, in the living room,' he whispers, giving a little bow of the head, his eyes closing momentarily behind a glint of steel-rimmed glasses, like a kindly psychoanalyst welcoming a new client. 'The social worker's with her at the moment. I don't suppose Maud will mind the two of you.'

Maud is sitting out of bed in an armchair, still wearing her cat-print pyjamas, looking around with a detached, slightly befuddled air. Beside her, on a hospital table, is a selection of the things she needs: tissues, beaker of tea, remote control, reading glasses, and a copy of Anna Karenina.

I introduce myself. When I shake hands with Maud she holds her hand out limply, looking up at me like someone who thinks they might still be asleep.

'I can't believe you're a hundred years old,' I say to her, sitting down opposite.

'Am I?' she says. 'Well, then. Neither can I.'

The social worker fills me in on the situation. Maud has Alzheimer's, but has been coping pretty well with care support and so on. Just recently there's been a bit of a decline, and people were worried.

'It doesn't look like an infection, so that's good,' says the social worker. 'Maud would like to stay in her home, but we've just been talking about that, and what we might be able to do to help.'

'I'm in your hands,' says Maud, then nods at Alan. 'You'll know what to do, won't you, dear?'

'It's whatever you want, Maud,' says Alan, smiling. 'But don't worry. Nothing's decided till it's decided.'

I carry out a quick set of observations whilst the social worker reads through the notes. Everything seems fine. Maud seems to be in rude health, considering her extreme old age.

'The thing that bothers me most,' says Maud, 'is I can't get up the stairs to look after Mum and Dad. And if I can't do it, who will?'

'By upstairs do you mean – upstairs? In the bedroom?'

'Where else would they sleep?'

'It's understandable that you're worried about them,' says the social worker, pausing a moment to choose her words. 'But I think they're safe now. I think they're pretty much at rest.'

'I know that!' says Maud. 'I'm a hundred years old! I'm not daft!'

'No,' says the social worker. 'You're certainly not.'

'It's just they're upstairs waiting for me, and I'm stuck down here, and I can't do anything about it.'

When it's time for me to go, Alan shows me to the kitchen door. I take this opportunity to ask him what he thinks about Maud. He stops to listen, adopting a thoughtful attitude, supporting the elbow of his right arm with the hand of his left, gently pinching his upper lip.

'I haven't met her before,' I tell him. 'So I don't know how much of this is new.'

'You mean this thing about her parents?'

'Has she talked about them before?'

'Off and on,' he says. 'I know how it sounds, but I suppose there are two ways of looking at it. One is that it's all just a symptom of her cognitive decline, some organic disease and so on. The other is to say that perhaps, yes, she can actually see her parents. You might think it odd to hear me say that; other people, in other cultures, with certain religious beliefs, would probably understand it quite well. You see, it's been my experience in circumstances like this that people nearing the end of life are – how shall I put this? – met?'

'That's certainly a different way of looking at it.'

'It is, isn't it!' he says, brightly, patting me on the shoulder. 'Now then. Good to see you, and thank you so much for coming!'

I walk over the road to my car and throw my bags in the boot. When I turn round to look, Alan's still there, watching me from the kitchen door.

I wave.

He waves back, then turns and goes inside.

For the life of me, I can't help glancing up at the bedroom window.

I come back the next day with Stacy, one of the physios. Stacy is exactly the kind of person you'd want to have with you in a haunted house. She may be small, but she has big feet, a disproportionately loud voice, and a vigorous, open-faced, square-shouldered approach to things. I can imagine her standing in the middle of a dark room, ghosts swirling round her, then planting her bag on the floor, clapping her hands and shouting: Right! Just because you've been dead two hundred years, doesn't mean you can fly around with bad posture. So straighten yourselves up, settle down, stop messing about and we'll see what we can do to help.

Stacy listens carefully when I tell her about what happened last time, the whole 'ghostly parents asleep upstairs waiting for their daughter' deal, and also about what her next of kin, Alan, had to say about it.

'Okay,' she says. 'Fine. But you do know that Maud spent many years looking after her parents? So I don't think it's all that surprising she's a bit muddled with the timings. I hardly know what day of the week it is myself, and I'm supposed to be young and fit.'

'No. I suppose – when you put it like that.'

She re-shoulders her rucksack, reaches up, and knocks so firmly with the rapper on the door it makes me think of Jack from Jack and the Beanstalk, knocking on the door of the giant's castle. Alan appears, still wearing the same Nordic sweater, shirt and tie, his goatee beard as perfectly groomed as a chin dipped in silver paint.

'Good to see you!' he whispers, shaking our hands. 'Thanks so much for coming.' He shows us in.

Maud is in the hospital bed in the living room, as before. If anything she seems in better form, alert and smiling, with that copy of Anna Karenina on her lap.

'Ah!' she says. 'Here comes the cavalry!' putting the book aside.

Maud has stopped being able to stand with assistance and transfer to the commode. There doesn't seem to be any infection or other organic reasons why she shouldn't be able to do this. And she certainly has the strength. When we've lowered the bed and raised the backrest, she swings her legs over the edge ready for the off. It's just – that's as far as she gets. Stacy is great at clearly and firmly describing what Maud needs to do to stand up, even sitting next to her at one point and demonstrating – but Maud just can't translate it into action. She keeps putting her feet too far out in front, and then waggling them up and down on the carpet, like a child splashing her feet in a puddle.

'It's no good!' she says. 'I'm falling!'

We persevere for as long as we can, but it's a game of diminishing returns. The more we try, the more anxious Maud becomes, until her efforts to stand are such an approximate and off-kilter thing, leaning back against our hands, the zimmer frame lifting off the carpet, that we have to accept defeat, and help her back to bed. It's strange to see how well she lifts her legs back onto the mattress and snuggle down again. Strength is certainly not the issue.

'It's definitely a confidence thing,' says Stacy, snapping off her gloves. 'Which isn't any less incapacitating, of course.'

'No, of course,' says Alan. 'But what's to be done?'

Stacy shrugs.

'Seems a shame to be thinking about hoisting. But other than that I suppose it's bed care and some gentle encouragement to overcome the block.'

'You see that woman over there,' says Maud, pulling the bedclothes up to her neck, and then pointing straight in front of her. For a second I wonder if it's another ghost – until I realise she means the sideboard facing her, and an ornate, silver frame in the centre of it. 'This one?' I say, going over to take a closer look. It's a sepia photograph of a young girl standing on a dark, southern English beach. She's dressed in a billowing white dress and enormous circular brimmed hat, which she holds on her head with one hand as she squints off into the distance. 'That's my mother,' says Maud. 'Now she'd have known what to do.'

꿍

Charles Court. Sounds like a tabloid headline but it's actually one of the smartest addresses in town. Even the approach is elegant: a shallow arrangement of steps and brass handrails, a decorative filigree canopy, wide, brass-handled glass doors, and swirling blue and white paisley tiling right and left – so that the whole thing looks more like the entrance to an expensive hotel than an apartment block.

I've actually come here to see two patients – a retired doctor with back pain on the sixth floor, and a newly catheterised patient on the fourth. I buzz the guy on the fourth, figuring I'll work my way up, just as a snappily dressed elderly man carrying a deli bag walks up the steps towards me.

'Excuse me, sir,' he says. 'Are you here to see Doctor Richards? I'm his friend and colleague, Doctor Samuels.'

'Nice to meet you,' I say, holding out my hand. He gives me the deli bag, which confuses me. We shake hands. I give him the bag back. Which confuses him. 'Thank you,' he says, immediately turning to walk back down the steps.

'Aren't you going to see your friend?' I say.

'What? Oh – yes! Yes, of course!'

He walks back up the steps, just as my patient answers the intercom.

'Dr Samuels here,' says Doctor Samuels, leaning pass me to answer in a gruff, doctorly kind of way.

'Who?' says my patient.

'It's okay,' I tell him. 'It's Jim, from the Rapid Response.'

'With a doctor?'

'No. He's visiting a friend. Another doctor.'

'Oh,' says my patient. He mutters something. The door buzzes. We both go into the lobby.

'Yes, yes,' says Doctor Samuels. 'Of course, we trained together,

Doctor Richards and I. Saint Bartholemew's, London. Nineteen fifty-nine! Sixty years ago!'

He shakes his head sadly.

'I'm seeing a patient on the fourth,' I tell him. 'But it won't take long and I'll be up to see Doctor Richards in about half an hour. Will you still be there, d'you think?'

'Yes, yes!' he says. 'Now look. I want to thank you for all the marvellous work you do. It's simply wonderful. We're very lucky to have you.'

'You're welcome.'

'I'm a doctor, too, you know. Well – retired! I've had my share of home visits, I can tell you!'

'I bet you have!'

'Oh my goodness, yes! I've been everywhere, seen everything and all stops in between. So I know what you're up against and I thank you most sincerely for the trouble you go to. It's much appreciated!'

'Pleasure!'

We walk together across the thickly carpeted lobby to the lift. I push the button. The doors slide open.

The lift is tiny – a sign of how old the place is, I would think. Dr Samuels is a portly guy in a huge mohair coat. He's even wearing some kind of panama hat with a brim. In fact, if he hadn't said he was a doctor I'd probably guess he was a Mafia Don. With all the bags I'm carrying, it's going to be quite a struggle for us both to fit in. For a second I'll think I'll take the stairs, but then Dr Samuels says: 'After you.'

'Well I'm getting out on the fourth and you want the sixth so maybe you should go first.'

'Please,' he says, pressing his eyes shut and gesturing to the lift. 'I insist.'

It's easier just to go along with it, so I say thank you and get in, putting my bags on the floor. Dr Samuels follows on, and we end up almost nose to nose. The doors slide shut, and for a moment we stand there, Dr Samuels with his eyes shut, breathing so heavily I'm worried he's fallen asleep.

'Excuse me...' I say, struggling to reach around him to press the buttons.

'Not at all! Not at all!' he says, still with his eyes shut.

The lift judders up.

'Ninety fifty-nine!' I say, to make conversation. 'That's a long time ago.'

'Yes,' he says. 'That's when I went to medical school to start my medical training, you know.'

'Is it?' I say. 'Amazing!'

'That's where we met, of course. Dr Richards and I.'

'At Barts.'

He opens his eyes.

'Yes!' he says. Why? Were you there, too?'

'Just a lucky guess.'

The door slides open.

'Well. This is me,' I say.

'Thank you,' he says, but even though I pick my bags up, he makes no effort to move. The doors slide shut again and we carry on up to the sixth.

'Here we are!' I say as positively as I can when the lift doors open again.

This time Dr Samuels does reverse out. I walk with him across the hallway to Dr Richard's flat, just to make sure he gets there safely. I don't want to be there when the door opens, though, because it'll be embarrassing to have to explain why I'm not coming in just yet. My other patient is expecting me. I've confused things enough as it is.

'I'll be back up in a minute,' I say, heading for the stairs.

'Why? Where are you off to?'

'Down to the fourth,' I say.

'Marvellous!' he says. 'Well. Lovely to see you!'

He makes no move to ring or knock, but I hope for the best and leave him to it.

When I turn to look for the last time, he's still standing there, idly rocking backwards and forwards. I wave, and he waves back with the hand holding the deli bag. Seems surprised to see it. Looks inside. Rummages around. Pulls out a sandwich. Starts eating it.

❧

'Is that a bird in the corner?'
  'A bird?'
  'A blackbird. Or a rat. Could be a rat. Something.'
  I go over to check, cautiously moving junk around.
  'No. Nothing here.'
  'Oh. I thought I saw something.'
  I put the junk back.
  'Do you think you might be hallucinating?'
  'No, no! I definitely saw it. This place – I don't know. Sometimes things just come in the door.'
  I don't know what to think. Steve's had a recent history of infection, and he certainly doesn't take care of himself, with his heavy drinking, his poor diabetes control, and the general state of his flat. But despite all this his obs are normal, and – so far at least – he's been pretty rational. And he's certainly right about the place. A tenement block you could use as a film set for the roughest quarter of New Orleans, with a dark, central courtyard, an old tree in a ruined brick planter, and all around rising up six storeys a crumbling iron fire escape.
  'Anyway. I wouldn't go to hospital, Jim. Not even if I was dying.'
  'Oh? Why's that?'
  'My son! I haven't seen him for ten years and he turns up yesterday.'
  'Wow! That's great!'
  'Yeah. He's off with his mates the other side of town. I 'spect I'll see him later.'
  There's a map of the world pinned to the wall above Steve's bed. He tells me about his life as the skipper of a yacht, sailing the world, working as a commercial diver, navigating the oceans through a haze

of booze, smoke and other substances until unexpectedly running aground in a wheelchair in this godforsaken flat.

'I've been through storms like you wouldn't believe. End of the World type storms. Did you know hurricanes give birth to tornadoes?'

'Do they?'

'I've seen it. The Devil's spawn. Evil snakes, twisting you into knots. I was always lucky, though. I've got a strong stomach. And better than that – a strong grip!'

Later that day, back at the hospital, his blood results come in – as bleak a set of figures as the worst severe weather warning. I book him an ambulance to go to hospital, and then call him to give him the news.

'I won't go without seeing my son,' he says.

'Can't you call him on his mobile?'

'I haven't got any credit on my phone, and he's left his at home.'

'I could call his landline and leave a message.'

'He lives in El Salvador.'

'Still, I could try...'

He gives me the number, but the number's unobtainable.

I ring Steve back and tell him what I think.

'The ambulance are on a two-hour response,' I tell him. 'So there's time. I'm not going to stand the ambulance down though, Steve, because your blood results are so out of whack I couldn't be responsible for that. Fingers crossed your son turns up between now and then. But your health's the most important thing.'

'I don't care about that,' he says. 'I'm not going anywhere till I've seen my son again.'

A little later I ring the hospital to check he went in. There's no record, so I ring Steve to find out what happened. When he answers the phone he sounds loud and emphatic, like he's speaking in the middle of a storm. I wonder if he's been drinking.

'No, Jim! He didn't show up!' he bellows. 'But even if he had I couldn't possibly go now.'

'Why's that?'

'It's all these kids.'

163

'What d'you mean? What kids?'

'All these seven-year-olds! Their mum's just dumped them here. And it's kinda weird, Jim – you know? Because they've done that thing kids do these days. They've painted their faces yellow and black. Fierce stripes, y'know! Like wasps...!'

I ring ambulance control again. Get the response time upgraded to immediate.

The living room is as brilliantly lit and formally arranged as the opening scene in a play. A man and a woman sitting side by side on the two-seater sofa in the bay window, stage left; me with my folder on my lap on a matching armchair just downstage from them, and then an elderly woman stage right, the focus of attention, sitting on a dining chair turned sideways to the table, her hands neatly folded in her lap. A bright and pleasant room, crowded bookshelves, pictures on the walls, a giant fern in a green pot, and a plain-framed mirror over the mantelpiece casting back that light pours in through the windows.

And if it was a scene from a play, the director might well decide to hold it there, curtain up, and not have anyone speak their lines for a beat or two, giving the audience time to settle, take it all in, and wonder about the four characters. What assumptions might they make?

They'd know I was official, and not just from the obvious stuff, the uniform and lanyard, bag and folders. They'd probably think there was something a little self-conscious about the way I was sitting, a conciliatory duck of the head, maybe, a professional sharing of attention between the other three. They'd think the other man was a relative, the son, no doubt. He's the right age, of course, but he looks like someone who's spent a lot of time in this room, one way or another. And the way he massages his hands and jogs his knee up and down. He looks like someone who's been brought here over some distance, at some inconvenience, still wearing the suit he was in when he took the call. A nice, professional son, then, worn down by circumstances he finds more difficult because they're out of the normal run of things, and hard to quantify in the usual way. The woman sharing the sofa is sitting so close to him they must be in a relationship. There's something resolutely straight-backed about her posture, the encouraging smiles she shares around the room, something about the way they are together that suggests long conversations and negotiations. They've arrived at a decision – he, more reluctantly – resolved to face it, shoulder to shoulder. The elderly woman has a bewildered look, a vagueness that's in strange contrast to the sharp delineation of everything else, as if the bright sunlight flooding the stage is causing her to lose definition rather than gain it.

'Tell me about the whole bath thing,' I say. 'I didn't get the whole story.'

'Well it does sound a bit crazy, even to me,' says Helen, the elderly woman. 'You see – I took a bath as I usually do in the evening, but then I blacked out, and it was some time before I was found.'

'How long?'

'Three days.'

'That is a long time.'

'Yes. It is.'

'Was the bath filled with water? You were lucky not to drown.'

'No. The water had gone.'

'Who drained it?'

'It must have been me, although I don't remember.'

'Three days in a bath! I'm surprised you didn't freeze.'

'It's a warm flat.'

'When did you regain consciousness?'

'The whole thing's blurry. I'm not really sure.'

'It's perhaps a strange question to ask, and I'm sorry for asking it – but had you been incontinent?'

'No, I hadn't.'

'So you passed out in the bath. Came round at some point. And then couldn't get out of the bath. Is that right?'

'I suppose so. Although it sounds pathetic when you put it like that.'

'Who found you?'

'Maria, the cleaner. She comes every Wednesday morning.'

'And did she call the ambulance?'

'Yes.'

'And they took you to hospital?'

'They did. And I had a whole series of tests. The works. And all they found wrong with me was a silly little cut on my toe. Would you like to see it?'

'Maybe in a minute or two.'

'I don't know how I did it. Probably on the tap, I should think.'

She looks at her son, Matthew, who sits on the sofa with his knee jogging up and down. Matthew's German wife, Helga, smiles brightly back at Helen.

'We will get things sorted,' Helga says. 'Don't worry.'

'Absolutely!' I say, flicking through the discharge summary, at the normal blood results and scans and so on, the recommended follow-ups. 'We'll figure something out.'

'I do hope so,' says Helen. 'It's all a bit of a drama, I'm afraid.'

9: Holding On

Malcolm doesn't have a phone. Not one that works, anyway. So all you can do is pitch up and hope for the best.

It's a fair bet he'll be in, though. For one reason or another he's had a series of falls – getting dizzy and going over at the bus stop, the queue at the post office, the supermarket. They've put him through the usual tests, given him a pacemaker, a range of medication, a walking stick. He's been to countless follow-up appointments (falling over on at least two of them). He's had a new hip. If you x-rayed his arm you'd see two plates and a line of screws. All in all, he's a walking (and falling) phenomenon. All they can really do now is adjust his meds from time to time, and maybe dress him like an American football player when he wants to go out.

'Come on in, why dont'cha!' he says when I knock on his open door.

He's bent over a boiled egg and crumpet, working away at it, his good elbow pointed straight up.

'Lovely!' he says, leaning back and wiping his chin. 'Now,' he says, waggling the eggy spoon in my direction, 'you can't do no better than an egg in the morning!'

These days Malcolm's flat is pretty down-at-heel, a settled and claggy sediment over every surface. Despite his straitened circumstance he declines all offers of help, though.

'I keep myself to myself,' he says. 'I don't do too bad.'

There are two black and white pictures on the wall behind him: Malcolm as a young man in the army. The first picture is of his unit, posing in full uniform in four rows; the second is a blow-up of the same picture, zooming in on Malcolm and the guys on either side. It's hard to see any likeness, though. Both pictures are so faded, it's disconcertingly like someone's dressed a row of mannequins in uniform, the peaked caps emphasising the blankness of their faces.

'I've jes' got to nip down to the laundry room,' he suddenly announces. 'You don't mind, d'you? Only the other fellas'll be gurnin' on about it.'

Before I can even offer to go for him – it's down two flights of stairs after all – he's pushed himself up from the armchair and set off.

'I'll come with you,' I say, hurrying after.

At least he lets me go down the stairs first.

When I take his bed clothes out of the dryer they're so hot I have to juggle them around.

'Done!' he says, slamming the dryer door in a blast of superheated, fabric-conditioned air. 'C'mon, fella!'

And we're off again.

He nods at the manager's door.

'Furloughed,' he says. 'Alright for some.'

'You can pause on the landing,' I say, chasing after him back up the stairs, almost tripping on the bottom sheet. 'There's no rush.'

He waves his hand in the air – which I'd rather he'd use to hold on to the rail.

'Feck it. If I go, I go,' he says. 'You can catch me in the sheets.'

Back in the flat, he tells me to dump the stuff on a chair by the bed. It's only then I notice his bed is heaped up with what looks like skeins of shredded cotton. It reminds me of the bedding my hamster used to have, how he'd scuffle it all up and then bury himself in the middle.

'Are you sure you wouldn't want someone to look in on you, Malcolm?' I say. 'We could get you some new bedding, if you'd like?'

'That's kind, but I'm okay,' he says, throwing himself down into the armchair again. 'Phew! That little jaunt took it out of me. You're spinning like a regular Father Christmas!'

'Father Christmas? Why? Does he spin?'

Malcolm rests his head back and closes his eyes.

'I don't know, fella,' he says. 'I don't know. It certainly looks that way to me now.'

The cautionary note on Maria's record was plain enough.

Naturist.

No exclamation point or any other modifier. Naturist. Just that. A succinct alert, short but informative.

I think about those signs you see on beaches sometimes: Clothes may not be worn beyond this point. It doesn't worry me, though. And I suppose it's good to get a heads up.

What it doesn't say – and which, in the end, is vastly more relevant – is that Maria likes to live in the dark.

'Mind yourself,' says her husband, John, a large, wild-haired man who holds the flat door open and makes an arch with his arm for me to duck under. Leaving the well-lit shared hallway to enter their grotto of inky black is something of an act of faith, only made possible by the thought that John surely HAS to be standing on the floor and not hovering like a malevolent angel over a chasm.

I feel my eyes widen as I struggle to adjust. The absence of light wouldn't be so bad if the place was clear. As it is, I bark my shins a few times and stumble over – what I take to be – a mobility scooter, a box of junk and either a grandfather clock or a coffin.

'Careful,' says John. 'D'you need a little light there?'

'Would be good.'

'Okay then.' He snaps a switch, and a few, long seconds later a tentative orange glow emanates from a silk covered lamp.

'Energy saving,' he says.

'Thanks.'

Still, it's better than nothing, just enough to illuminate the room in front of me where Maria is waiting on the sofa. At least naked she's easier to make out, the mass of her large pale body accentuated by the square of white muslin she's draped over her middle. She's like the Venus of Willendorf, on the sofa, with a remote.

'Sorry, pet,' she says, turning off the TV and then tossing the remote to one side. 'Have a seat.'

'Don't worry,' I tell her. 'I've got to keep moving or I'll grind to a halt.'

I think about the torch I've got in my bag, and wonder about getting it out.

She shrugs, adjusts her square, then sits staring into the blank TV screen opposite. I look into it, too – at our faint reflections, me in my uniform, Maria naked on the sofa, the two of us caught like mysterious phantoms in the depths of a scrying mirror.

'How long have you lived here?'

'Ooh – I don't know. I should think about sixty years or more,' says Thomas. 'We moved when we had Lily, and I'd got that new job. D'you remember, Lucy?'

'Of course I remember!' says Lucy, rearranging a napkin on her lap. 'I was here, wasn't I?'

'Sixty years,' says Thomas, absorbing Lucy's tetchiness with a wistful shake of his head and then a sudden, gaping smile, the kind you might see on a ventriloquist's dummy. 'Long enough!' he says.

It's a beautiful old cottage – or used to be. Could be again, with a little work. Emptying out all the clutter, ripping out what remains of the fixtures and fittings, stripping back the plaster to the bricks, taking up the floor, rewiring, new doors and windows. New roof, come to that. Redecorating throughout. Cutting back the garden, and so on. An album of Before and After photographs. These things take a little imagination, but totally worth it if you can see beyond the mess. Clink, clink. Cheers!

Thomas and Lucy wouldn't feature in any of the quotes, of course, even if the builders were game, and had a few geriatricians, cosmetic surgeons and orthopaedic consultants on the team. Because it goes without saying that the same passage of years that wreaked such damage on this house hasn't spared the occupants, and whilst ancient buildings can be straightened out with hard work and a certain amount of cash, the same can't be said of the people who live in them.

'Push that button – no! That one!' says Thomas, leaning out to interfere with Lucy's attempts to operate the riser-function of her chair.

'Let me do it! Let me do it…!' says Lucy, wresting it away from him and getting in a muddle. The back of the seat goes down and the footrests shoot out. 'Blast!' she says, and promptly turns the whole thing off.

They have carers three times a day – once to get them up and dressed, once to give them lunch and prepare some cling-filmed sandwiches for tea, and once to put them to bed. Although I have to say it's looking pretty much as if the 'bed' aspect has gone by the board. They're sleeping in their chairs full-time now, and only getting up to stagger precariously through the jumble of everything to a commode.

At first it seems like a pretty sad kind of existence, and I can't help feeling sorry for them. Wouldn't it be better if they sold up and moved into a nursing home? Somewhere with staff on hand to keep an eye on them? To wash, dress and feed them, and keep them warm (not that this place is cold – they have a free-standing oil-filled radiator in the middle of the room, on full). I'm sure they could sit next to each other somewhere, either in their own room or in the lounge? Because no-one could say they were remotely safe in this place. A small stack of ambulance sheets is a testament to the increasing number of falls they're having.

But they don't strike me as unhappy. The bickering isn't unpleasant or aggressive; more the sniping of two caged creatures, fussing over the minutiae of their shrunken existence. I wonder how well they'd fare if they were removed from this place, even taking into account the trip hazards and the damp and the dodgy electrics. I wouldn't be surprised if they faded away the moment they were helped to a couple of comfortable chairs, in a wide and well-lit room, with a television, and a trolley doing the rounds at half-past ten, and three.

'Give it here… look! You've turned the damned thing off!'

Thomas tries to snatch the remote, but it's like watching a tortoise make a swipe for another tortoise's lettuce leaf.

'Ha!' says Lucy. Then after glaring at him triumphantly, she slowly presses it up to her nose to figure it out.

You wouldn't think people actually lived on this street. It's one of the main thoroughfares, an artery of urban bustle, crowds spilling over the pavements day and night, drinking in the pubs and cafes, streaming in or out of the concert venue, staring in the windows of the chi-chi boutiques, taking selfies outside the old theatre, or crowding round the buskers who work the passing trade on the pedestrian cut-throughs. The street heads up at a shallow incline, diverging endlessly left and right, then gradually thins, and quietens, until it runs out of energy at the top, where a main road cuts across it at right angles, running from the station to the sea. Here the shops are more down-at-heel. There's a secondhand camera shop, an antique clothes shop, a tailoring and alteration shop, a shop for rent, all of them weathered and worn, their wooden facades peeling. The person who did the display in the window of the antique clothes shop – how long ago? – has opted for a nightmarishly whimsical look: a stuffed fox head tied into a hacking jacket; some tackle lying around, a few vacant toys, as if they'd given up trying and taken to lure customers in with appalled terror instead. I wonder if there's anyone in the shop at all. Maybe they're just behind the netting, holding their breath, staring at me as I cup my hand on the glass to see better.

Mr Lake lives in the flat above the tailoring shop next door. There's a young woman sitting in the shop window, dreamily needling some trousers draped on her lap. She pauses with the needle in mid-air as I fetch the key from the keysafe and turn to open the side door. I smile and nod but she doesn't acknowledge me; in fact, I don't even see her lower the needle as I push the side door open.

The hallway is dark and cramped, the only light coming from a yellowing square of glass at the far end, and a single, winking point of red from the console of the electric scooter on charge. I can't see a switch for any hall light, and there's no room for me to put my bag down and find my torch, so instead I wait a minute until my eyes have adjusted, then slowly creep forwards past the scooter and piles of junk, onto the sagging carpet of the stairs, and head up.

'Hello? Mr Lake? It's Jim – from the hospital.'

There's a TV playing in one of the rooms overhead, a rowdy studio debate, raucous shouting and applause – which somehow makes the place feel quieter.

'Hello?'

A toilet with no door on the first little landing, a twist to the left, a galley kitchen on the right with a glimpse of stacked plates and bulging plastic bags, and then up onto the top landing, where a heavy curtain has been nailed across a doorway.

'Mr Lake?'

I hook the curtain aside.

Mr Lake is sitting on a high-backed chair, surrounded by boxes and cabinets, piles of old Picture Post and Hobbycraft magazines, crates of clocks and Teasmades and novelty telephones. It's difficult enough for me to find a way through all the mess, so I can't imagine how Mr Lake manages it. But then, no doubt, he's used to it all and it fits him pretty well, like a hermit crab making its shell from a tin can or a discarded doll's head.

I'm here to dress a wound on his leg. It's not easy, setting up a sterile field, though. I have to move a few things.

'Temporarily!' I tell him. 'If I'd had a pound for every time I'd said temporarily....'

'You'd have five pounds fifty!' he says.

'No doubt.'

We chat whilst I set up. He tells me about his life. How he used to be an engineer.

'I was always good with my hands,' he says. 'Taking things apart, putting them back together, that kind of thing.'

'That's a great skill to have.'

'It kept me fed and watered.'

I glove up.

'Any family in the area...?' I ask as I lean in to remove the old dressing. The smell is gacky – the cloyingly sweet smell of decay.

'No. No family,' he says, watching me drop the filthy dressing into the waste bag. 'I was married for a while. But she left. Ran off with the best man. And one day he dropped dead in the garden. So she hanged herself.'

'Oh – I'm sorry,' I say, changing my gloves. 'That's terrible.'

'Ah. Well,' he says. 'She was always a bit up and down.'

When I've finished the dressing and I'm ready to go, I notice some framed pictures on the wall behind the TV.

'Is that you?' I say, pointing at the picture of a smiling young man in a smart suit and waistcoat, holding a scowling baby up to the camera.

'No! That's my mother!' he says.

'Your mother? What? This one?'

'Where are my glasses...?' says Mr Lake. He grumbles and fumbles around his chair, the glasses magically appear in his hand, he hooks them over his ears, then screws up his face and leans forward.

'Oh. Yes. You're right. That's me,' he says.

'Who's the baby?'

'That one? No idea.'

Amongst all the other portraits is one of a young woman in a floppy white hat and wide-collared raincoat. It's a posed, three-quarter shot, the woman staring sleepily off to the right, her eyes heavy, her mouth slightly open. The odd thing is, she has her right hand raised in mid-air, palm down, off to the side at shoulder height, as if she's pushing through invisible undergrowth, or maybe working a marionette whose strings she'd dropped but didn't think anyone would notice.

'That's her,' says Mr Lake. 'That's my wife. She made that coat. The day I took the photo we'd gone out for something to eat. We were sitting in the cafe, and the owner of a fancy boutique came over, and he said Where did you get that coat? And she said I made it. So he said Why don't you come and work for me! We need people like you.'

'And did she?'

'No,' says Mr Lake. 'She didn't.'

❧

Jack is sitting slumped on the edge of his bed, a huge brown dressing gown draped over his shoulders.

'I'll make more sense when I put my teeth in,' he says. 'Get 'em for me, would you? Go through to the kitchen. Hard left. Over to the sink. On the window ledge, by the soap dish. You'll find 'em there. Give 'em a rinse and I'll bung 'em in.'

It's the fourth or fifth trip I've made to the kitchen. First it was a cup of tea. Then it was his slippers. He wanted a knife to open the letters I'd pulled out of the letterbox – but not the knife I brought through. He wanted his frame....

I find the teeth, soaking in an old yogurt pot. They look a little scummy, so I run them under the tap.

'That's the ones!' he says, reaching out for them. 'Jes' a minute.'

He puts them in – an extraordinary process, his wrinkled mouth gabbling round the plates. It's like watching an octopus trying to crack an oyster. Finally he gets the teeth into position, then hands me the yogurt pot again.

'Done,' he says. 'Put that back.'

I don't mind his bossiness. There's something about the way he gives all these orders, directly and without an edge, that makes it entertaining. Anyway, he's had a hard time lately. Not only has he fallen over twice – once in the surgery, once at home – but now his boiler's broken and there's no heating or hot water.

'Never mind that,' he says. 'Set that sofa back over there, would you? Not there. There!'

He used to be a motor mechanic and I can quite imagine him up to his knotty elbows in grease, a fag in the corner of his mouth, shouting something across a garage in the nineteen-fifties. Something about a wrench.

175

He's got so many wounds on his arms and hands it takes me a while to check them all and renew the dressings.

'There!' I say at last, tossing the last of the wrappers in the rubbish bag and peeling off my gloves. 'That'll get you through the MOT.'

'You think?' he says. 'We'll see!'

I take the trash out and bring him another cup of tea.

'Put it there,' he says. 'Now – move the table closer. That's it! Y'know – them girls'll miss me down the surgery. I was supposed to go there today with my feet. You wait till they hear what happened,' he says, wrapping his horrible brown dressing gown more tightly around himself. 'They'll piss 'emselves laughing.'

His old friend Sally has been keeping an eye on things, but she's in her eighties, hasn't been round in a while.

'I don't suppose I'll see her for a few weeks,' he says. 'If ever. Did I tell you how we met?'

I'm writing the notes up, so I'm only half-listening when he tells me the story, a long and complicated affair that mostly seems to focus on a guy called Barry. I lose the thread and ask him who Barry is.

'Oh never mind,' he says. 'It was a long time ago.'

The last thing I do before I go is make Jack's bed up. These days he's sleeping downstairs on a rickety put-you-up, something he's adamant he doesn't want changing.

'I'm used to it,' he says. 'I know its ways.'

I make the bed as well as I can, shaking out the duvet, plumping the pillows, smoothing the bottom sheet, lining up the duvet and tucking it in the wall-side, putting his favourite tartan blanket neatly over the bottom half of the bed, then turning back the near corner so it's ready. When I'm done, I stand at the head end and salute.

'Military man?' he says.

'No,' I tell him. 'I thought about it once, but I'm no good at taking orders.'

Craig is a heavy-set young guy with even heavier-set eyes. He's sitting in an armchair almost completely walled-in with books, some open, some being used as improvised tables for his bottles of Dr Pepper and No Sugar Sprite. Books on the occult, alien conspiracy theories, tarot. Books on the history of the horror film, on special effects, warcraft, sorcery, sex magic. Books on PHP, C#, Javascript. And, weirdly, a book on rabbits.

'I've come to take your blood,' I say.

'Whatever,' he says.

He's extraordinary. A long, black pencil moustache trailing down either side of an equally long goatee, giving him the look of a sleepy catfish – except a catfish that had spent as much time in the piercing and tattoo parlours as the mud at the bottom of the lake. His tattoos are amazing. Full sleeve canvases of skulls and roses and ivy leaves, swords, flames, goblins, and here and there a portentous Latin phrase in gothic print.

'Good luck finding a vein,' he says, extending his right arm and resting it on the top of some books.

He's right. It's going to be tricky. Normally if a patient is large and you can't see the veins, you can work by feel. In Craig's case, the intricate lines of ink have raised the skin, so what feels like a vein is actually the stem of a rose or the ribbed hilt of a dagger. I'm prodding around for quite a while. To pass the time we talk about tattoos. I show him mine, the Tree of Life I had done on the top of my left arm. He's polite about it but doesn't seem that impressed.

'There's a lot of people doing it now,' he says. 'Most studios can sort you out with that kind of thing.'

'I went for hand-poked,' I tell him. 'I don't know why particularly. I liked the idea that's how people tattooed themselves before electricity.'

'Yeah,' he says. 'The whole primitive thing.'

'I want to get another one, a bit lower down. It's quite addictive.'

'Tell me about it,' he says.

'There! What about there? That feels like something.'

He shrugs. 'If you think. I'm okay with it.'

Amazingly, the blood flows immediately.

'I can't believe it!' I tell him when I'm done, withdrawing the needle and taping on some gauze. 'I wasn't at all confident with that one.'

'It's the book you were leaning on,' he says, holding it up so I can read the cover.

Divination for Beginners.

Then closing his eyes and smiling, he slowly strokes his feelers, like that was his plan all along.

Talking to Mr Carrington on the phone, I imagine him to be something like Mr Banks from Mary Poppins, sitting in a wing back armchair by an open fire, glass of brandy in one hand, phone in the other, hospital discharge summary on his tartan-rugged lap.

'It's the most extraordinary thing,' he says. 'And to cap it all I have to wear this blasted boot.'

'I'll be over in about half an hour.'

'Splendid! D'you know where I am?'

'Roughly. How far down is number seventy?'

'Stand in front of the old pub, turn to your right, stride up the hill three lampposts, turn and fire. Can't miss.'

'Great. See you shortly.'

'Righto. Let yourself in. You'll find me upstairs. Downstairs is rather out of bounds at the moment.'

I'm sorry to say that even Mary Poppins, with all her grit and sparkle and domestic magic, would take one look at number seventy, blush and pretend to have an appointment on the other side of town.

It's a deeply unprepossessing row, one house leaning against its neighbour up the hill like drunks on a tipping bench. Number seventy is probably the worst, with its gappy tiles, hanging gutterings, cracked windows, rotten fascias, peeling paint, and a malign-looking buddleia standing like a giant spider by the broken gate, arching its branches over the steps.

I don't open the door so much as lift it delicately to one side. In front of me is a damp and gloomy hallway, a precipitous flight of stairs.

'Up here!' shouts Mr Carrington.

'Okay...'

The stairs creak and give alarmingly. When I put out a hand to grab the rail, it wobbles with such a wormy shudder I decide to take my chances and pick my way spot to spot with my hands free.

Onto the landing, and another vista of neglect. Whole sections of wallpaper rolling off the walls. A scattering of junk. Skeins of old web. A spotted smell so rich you can hear it muttering.

'First door on your left,' says Mr Carrington. 'If there was a door.'

Astonishingly, someone's managed to cram a hospital bed into the room, squeezing it in at the only possible angle that could work. Behind it is a bookshelf filled with dusty books and crowned with a leather briefcase that looks like it's just been fished out of a pond.

'Good to see you!' says Mr Carrington.

We shake hands.

If this is Mr Banks, he's been marooned on an island for a good many years – which I suppose, in a way, he has. His mane of ash grey hair flows into an equally vast beard, so wild I only see he has a mouth when he laughs.

After my examination – which he passes easily, with nothing concerning in any of his observations – I try to talk to him as tactfully as I can about his circumstances, the trip hazards, the damp and so on. Each point he bats away with the practised ease of someone who's had the same conversation many times before.

'Don't worry. I'm quite used to it,' he says. 'Honestly. I'm quite happy as things are. Once my foot is better I'll be able to tootle down the shops as before. So long as someone can fetch me a few essentials in the meantime, I'll be absolutely fine.'

The room is freezing, though. When I tell him how worried I am about that he laughs.

'Oh for goodness sake!' he says, swatting the air between us. 'I like it cold. Always have. It keeps me sharp! And if I get a bit chilly – well! I've got my cosy.'

He roots around under his pillow, produces a filthy hat and pulls it over his head, squashing his hair out to the side.

'See?' he says. 'What d'you think?'

'Well. It certainly looks – warm.'

'Exactly!' says Mr Carrington, snatching it off again, his hair springing back. 'So there we are, then. Now. Let's talk about something else. Let's talk about you.'

I can see Jeremy through the window, sitting in an armchair in front of the television, his fingers laced across his bare chest, his eyes closed, the television bathing him in a flickering blue light. I watch for a moment, to make sure that he is actually breathing, and it's not some animating trick of the light. But then he squeezes his eyes and wrinkles his nose, and adjusts the position of his head on the cushion. I tap on the window again.

Even though the screen is facing away from me, I can tell it's an old David Niven film. That beautifully modulated, terribly sincere English accent. But you know, are you in love with anybody? No, no don't answer that…

'Jeremy? Jeremy! Can you come to the door? It's Jim, from the hospital.'

He doesn't respond. I knock again. When he seems to open one eye, I press my ID badge against the pane. It's no use. He sinks back into what now appears to be a determined kind of sleep.

Not that I'm keen to go in. I've already been warned to wear shoe covers, and I can see through the window that the accounts of rotting food and piles of rubbish were no exaggeration. Anyway, even if I hadn't seen the report, the windowsill would tell me all I needed to know. It's littered with the husks of flies, lying on their backs with their legs crimped up, so large I'm guessing they just dropped from the air and died from sheer luxuriousness, whilst around them, hyperactive amongst the webby detritus on the windowsill, a multitude of jumpy, crawly things, sensing fresh blood, are hurling themselves against the glass.

I take a step back, scratch my head, then try his mobile once again. I can hear it ringing somewhere amongst the trash, but it doesn't rouse him any more than my banging on the window.

Even though it looks from here as if he just doesn't want to acknowledge my presence, I can't rule out the possibility that he's unwell with a hypo or something. But just as I try the handle of the door to see if it's actually open, a woman coughs and says hello from the end of the path.

'Have you come to see Jeremy?'

'Yeah. I can see him sitting in his chair but he doesn't seem to want to come to the door.'

'I'm Sharon, his neighbour,' she says, holding out her hand. 'It's probably down to me that you've been called.'

'Oh?'

We chat in the cover of an overgrown buddleia.

'We've been increasingly worried about Jezza,' says Sharon. 'He's been on the slide for some time now, a good few years. Ever since Eric died. Then he lost his job, and things went from bad to worse. He hasn't put a foot outside the house in eight months or more. If it wasn't for us and number twenty, he'd have starved to death. He's skin and bone as it is. And his house. Well, I mean, my god...'

'I know. I can see through the window.'

'It's worse inside.'

'I've got shoe covers.'

'Yeah? I think you're gonna need something more than shoe covers. You need one of them biohazard suits you see in the films.'

She mimes one, holding her arms out to the side, rocking a little from side to side and puffing out her cheeks.

'I could totally use it,' I say. 'But I'll just have to make the shoe covers stretch.'

'Good luck with that.'

'What does his doctor say?'

'I mean – they have tried, bless 'em. But it's difficult. He was driving to the supermarket till recently.'

She turns to look at the wreck on the road outside the house, a mossy old Rover saloon, melting into its tires. 'Mind you,' she says, 'I'm glad he's done with all that. He was a menace. He used to go at five miles an hour, all the traffic building up behind him, going crazy. And he wouldn't park so much as randomly stop and get out. It's a shame. He used to be a nurse, funnily enough.'

I'm just about to ask Sharon some more questions when the front door opens and Jeremy pokes his head out.

'Ah! Hello Jeremy!' I say. 'Sorry to disturb you.'

'That's okay,' he says in a voice as smooth and dry as greaseproof paper. I can see from here how emaciated he is, the ribs and bumps and hollows of his torso a testament to years of self-neglect. He opens the door wider and smiles unexpectedly, with a flare of yellowing stumps

'How can I help?' he says.

The cottage that Jenny has shared with her mother for thirty years is a narrow, two-storey affair, squashed between its neighbours, a knocked-through living area at ground level, Jenny's bedroom and a spare room on the first, her mother's bedroom and the bathroom on the second, the whole thing connected by a staircase as bare and steep as a spinal column. Over the years the two of them have held onto everything that came their way – books, pictures, papers, nick-nacks, cables, lamps, linen, plates, cameras, typewriters, spools of thread, film, whatever – the whole lot either stuffed in carrier bags, strapped in old suitcases or packed in plastic crates, everything piled-up, stuffed-in, balanced-on, walled-up, to the extent that you turn round on the spot looking for somewhere to put your bags, complete a full circle, and end up standing there smiling bravely instead.

'I'm so sorry about the mess – I've been trying to have a bit of a tidy up since mummy became ill – well, I say ill – I should say iller – if that was a word – is that a word? – maybe I just invented a word! – because you know I'm not the full ticket myself – I'm half worn out – you should see me going up those stairs – on all fours half the time – like a goat! – well, not a goat, more like a monkey – a monkey with a bad back – you see, I had a cancer scare – I'm sixty after all – I suppose you've got to expect these things – it's a shock when they happen, though – don't get me wrong – you know about mummy's cancer, don't you? – riddled with it I shouldn't wonder – but she won't let them look – she won't listen to anyone – never has – look at this place! – but if I threw out one little scrap she'd know and have a fit – come in a bit, I need to lock the door behind you – I never know whether lifting the handle on its own is good enough – best not take chances...'

It's a test of spatial reasoning to figure out how Jenny is to get past me and my three bags of kit without one of us either burying ourselves, or both of us going outside and coming back in again in reverse order. Meanwhile, Jenny talks constantly through the whole, complex procedure. It strikes me that her conversation is a verbal representation of the house, lacking any kind of editing function, any random thought or memory as good as the next, no clear space, nothing to point. The stress of the situation doesn't help, of course. It sounds as if their relationship has been pretty difficult over the years. As Jenny's monologue continues, an image slowly develops behind it, like a Polaroid picture moving from ghostly impression to something more solid, something with colour and depth, a long face, thin lips, guarded expression.

'Straight up – right to the top – well, I SAY the top....we're coming, mummy!...'

Jenny follows behind, on all fours.

Tony has a range of character phones. Tweety Pie, Hello Kitty, Bugs Bunny and so on. All of them bravely maintaining their expressions beneath the same grimy brown patina that covers everything in the room. It's an astonishing thing, a dismal, bristling crust that wouldn't look out of place on the wreck of a ship at the bottom of the Atlantic. And if this was a ship, I'd guess, through the visor of my mask, that I'd swum into the nursery, because encircling the whole room are three shelves, each of which is packed full of toys and childish souvenirs of every description: elephants, camels, teddy bears and finger drums, Chad Valley projectors, unidentifiable figures in corroded snow globes, figurines in decaying boxes from shows I've never heard of – the whole, mouldering cargo merging one thing into another, in one great soup of neglect.

'Quite a collection you've got,' I say as I take his blood pressure.

'Inherited,' he sniffs. 'I had six relatives all die in the space of two years. I got rid of what I could. The rest just stayed.'

'I'm sorry.'

'It was a bad time that's for sure,' he says, rolling his sleeve down again. He coughs – such a sludgy sound it's hard to resist the idea that his lungs are coated in the same noxious matter as the rest of the room. 'I fell ill. And then my support worker died.'

'How awful!'

'He dropped dead in this room, right about where you're standing now.'

'Terrible. I feel awful. It's my breathing. I can't get my breath. And there's nothing worse, is there? Not breathing? I've been like it months. Ever since I come home. Ever since I had the fall. I was going out to the garage. I can't think why. A slipper come off and I missed the step. Went backwards. Right over the mobility scooter. Pulled a ladder down on top. I was stuck there ages. Calling for help. Brian come out, eventually. When he was hungry. He's no help. He's got dementia. He just stood looking at me from the step. What are you doing down there? he said. Then he went back inside. Six hours I was out there. In the freezing cold. The paramedics had a hell of a job. They had to use special equipment. Special blankets. Took me up the hospital. Found I'd broke three ribs. Caught pneumonia. Shocking state. Couldn't sleep. People dying all around. There was one on the right. I heard them work on her. I watched her legs kicking up and down. Course – it was no good. They called it a day and went. Only they didn't draw the curtains properly. I could still see her head on the pillow. All that long grey hair. I couldn't stop staring. I couldn't help myself. Eventually they showed up. The men in green. I heard them zipping up the bag. Wheeled her off. Later on I told the nurse. Why didn't you say anything? she said. We would've shut the curtains. But I didn't say anything, did I? I just sat there, staring. The long grey hair, hanging off the pillow like that. I went home the day after. But I can't stop thinking about it. The gap in the curtains. The hair on the pillow. I mean – what are you supposed to do with something like that?'

10: What a Performance

'Tell me about the squirrel.'

'It would never have happened if Sheila were still alive.'

'Was she good with squirrels?'

'She was good with everything. I'm lost without her. Lost and lonely.'

'I'm sorry to hear that.'

'It's not your fault.'

'So go on, then. What's all this about a squirrel?'

'I'd just got back from the shops. I opened the front door and came into the hallway, put the bag, leant the stick in the corner, turned round to close the door when I heard this little skittery noise from the bedroom. Hello I said. Who's there? Because I thought it might be a burglar. Which, in a way, it was. So I nudged forward a little bit, and there was the skittery noise again, and something falling over, like a glass. So I said Right! I'm calling the police – although the phone was in the kitchen, and anyway, to be honest with you, I had a feeling it was too small to be a burglar. More likely a cat or something. But you say stupid things when you're on your own, don't you? Sheila wouldn't have had none of that. She'd have marched right in there and sorted it out, burglar or otherwise. She was always the same, right from when we met. She weren't afraid of nothing, except maybe at the end, and that was different. That was more than anyone could've coped with. Anyway, there I was, standing in the hallway, wondering what to do, picking my stick up again and holding it out in front of me, when suddenly – wham! Out flies this squirrel. And I know I've probably remembered it all wrong, because it happened so quick, but I swear, this squirrel, he ran up the wall, across the ceiling, back down the other side, through my legs and out the front door. And I spun round on the spot to whack him one, and fell over, and I must've caught my head on the hall table, because next thing I know I'm sitting on the carpet covered in blood, and my daughter Carol's standing over me, and she's saying Oh my God, Dad. What happened to you? And I told her about the squirrel, and she told the paramedics, and now everyone thinks I'm this crazy old fool who got mugged by a squirrel. But I tell you what, they're not like they used to be. I remember when a squirrel would tiptoe up to you and maybe take a nut or two out your hand. Now they're just as likely to steal your car and burn your house down. But things change, I suppose. Life goes on. I just wish I was coping better.'

Muriel had a fall recently. She hurt her neck, so they put her in a support, a fat, white fabric affair that pushes her chin up and makes a presentation of her face, a modern riff on the Elizabethan ruff. Muriel doesn't look too happy about it. In fact, her expression is intensely mournful. You could draw her face pretty quickly as a series of downward curves: two for the eyes, two smaller ones for the nostrils, one big one for the mouth.

'I've popped in to see how you are, Muriel. And the physio asked me to give you this zimmer frame.'

'Oh yes?' she says, leaning forwards but not actually opening her eyes. 'Why would I want that, then? I've got my stick.'

'Your stick's great, but this is safer,' I say, slapping it twice, like some kind of dodgy market trader. 'They say you've had a few falls lately, Muriel, so hopefully this'll help.'

'Everyone's been so kind,' she says, turning away and heading back to the sofa. 'I don't know. I just don't know.'

The referral had come from the ambulance, but we've had plenty of follow-up calls, especially from the neighbours. They've seen her wandering outside the house at all hours, distressed, confused. At least now there are several people on the case – the GP, social services, mental health and other nurses. A night sitter has been booked to keep an eye on things tonight, but a decision will have to be made soon as Muriel isn't safe to be home alone.

I help her settle back on the sofa. I offer to make her a cup of coffee

188

and find some biscuits.

'You don't mind if I watch my quiz?' she says.

'Of course not.'

'I like my quizzes.'

'I bet.'

The TV is playing one of those afternoon shows where the set is so emphatically neon it makes you feel scratchy and slightly hysterical. I wouldn't be able to answer with my own name, let alone who played James Bond in Dr No. The quizzes always have to have a gimmick. This one seems to be about lists. The contestants answer questions on a subject, and either go through and win some money, or not. Warwick Davis presides over the whole thing with a smile as bright as his shirt.

'Let's play Lists!' says Warwick.

I escape into the kitchen.

It's so orderly in there I wonder whether this confusion is more an acute thing, or whether Muriel already has help of some kind. Everything's exactly where you'd expect it to be. Utensils hanging in height order from a rack. Chopping boards neatly aligned. There's even coffee in a jar marked 'Coffee'. When I fetch the milk out of the fridge, the souvenir magnets are all lined up in alphabetical order. There's a big ceramic bear on the counter. When I twist its head off I find it's filled with mini cookies. I grab out a handful, arrange them in a circle on a saucer, and take it all through on a tray decorated with kittens.

On the telly lights are flashing and klaxons sounding, so I'm guessing someone is going home empty-handed.

'There you go, Muriel!' I say, putting the coffee and biscuits on the table beside her. 'I'll just write up my notes in the folder then I'll leave you in peace.'

'Righto,' she says, tossing down the cookies one after the other, crumbs already sticking to the powdered hairs on her chin.

The yellow nursing folder is in the middle of a circular dining table on the far side of the room. There are no chairs round the table, except for a green plastic garden chair with a wooden box on it. The box has a brass plate – commemorating the ashes of her husband Frank who died just a couple of years ago. It's strange to see the box there. It's such a formal, substantial thing, like a miniature coffin. I wonder whether Muriel's taken it down from somewhere to clean it, or whether she moves it about and talks to it. I try to imagine how I'd feel, having it around the place, like I'd been interrupted on the way to the cemetery. Something like the cookie jar would be friendlier and less – well – jarring.

'Let's play Lists!' says Warwick.

Maud is watching 'Lawrence of Arabia' on a plasma TV screen so enormous you'd need a camel to get from one side to the other. She's sitting in a padded wheelchair, her bad right leg straight out on a leg support. It's a nice contrast, seeing Maud in her wheelchair like that, Peter O'Toole on his camel. I picture her tying her leg to the hump.

'Have you ever ridden one of those?' I ask her.

'No. But I went on the dodgems once.'

Maud's daughter Isabel is supposed to be meeting me here. She's already rung to apologise and say she'll be late, though. Apparently the taxi driver sat outside her house and didn't bother letting her know he was there.

Maud shakes her head.

'That's Isabel for you,' she says.

We've done all the medical stuff so there's nothing to do but wait. Isabel has some questions and concerns, so I need to hang on for a while.

'I hope she won't be long,' I say.

'She'll be twenty minutes,' says Maud. 'You can set your watch by it.'

We watch as Peter O'Toole and his guide draw water from a well in the middle of a vast expanse of desert. Suddenly they see a shimmering black shape in the distance. A mirage? What is it? The shape gets bigger. A figure on a camel, riding straight at them. The

Arab guide fetches out a rifle and takes aim. Peter O'Toole tries to stop him but it's too late. The approaching figure fires first; the guide drops to the sand, dead. Finally the figure arrives. It's Omar Sharif.

'Now there's a good-looking man,' says Maud, pushing herself more upright in the wheelchair. 'He can shoot me any day.'

'I've got a story about Omar Sharif,' I say.

'Oh yes?'

'My brother in law is Lebanese. Or was. He's dead now, unfortunately.'

It suddenly strikes me it's an odd thing to say. Do you stop being Lebanese just because you died? Maybe you do. Maybe that's death. You stop being anything.

'What did he die of?'

'Cancer.'

'Yes,' says Maud, flatly, as if she expected it all along.

'Anyway, he used to work in Maroush, a famous Lebanese restaurant on the Edgware Road.'

'I've heard of it, I think.'

'It's pretty swanky. Saad was the Head Waiter. One day Omar Sharif came in, surrounded by all these glamorous people. Saad went to take their order and settle them in, and Omar looked up at him and said: Would you like my autograph? And Saad said: No. Would you like mine?'

'I liked him in Doctor Zhivago,' says Maud. 'He was lovely in that.'

'I haven't seen that one.'

'No? You should.'

Me, Maud and Peter O'Toole watch Omar Sharif ride away on his camel.

The door bursts open. It's Isabel.

'So sorry about that!' she says. 'Stupid driver.'

❦

La Contessa is sitting in her riser recliner, one hand clapped over the business end of a cordless phone, the other held out to me – whether to shake or kiss, it's hard to tell.

Are you still there, Doctor? she shouts into the phone, flapping her free hand for me to come in and sit down somewhere, anywhere. Hello? No – that was the nurse. Come to sort me out, I should think. I should HOPE. Now – this really is the most awful bother I'm in. Those pills you gave me aren't doing the trick and I need something stronger. Something with a bit more of a kick. Mildred my domestic was telling me about the lovely liquid morphine she was given for her knee. She said she took a slug of it every time she had a twinge and it sorted her out nicely. I rather like the sound of that. So I'd be awfully grateful if you could see your way to organising that for me........ Well, I'm hardly like to do that, am I? I haven't moved from the chair in the last day or so.....No, not even for that..... which is why I'm rather hoping this kind nurse may have brought a special something to help with that aspect. (She glances over at me, raises her eyebrows, and nods.) Yes, she says into the phone, he just made a gesture to indicate that he HAS brought something.......Okay Doctor? Thank you, Doctor. I'll say goodbye for now, and I look forward to seeing you soon. Lovely. Cheerio.

She presses the phone off in an overly forceful way – more like she's grinding out a revolting bug with her thumb – then places it on the table of things next to her chair, and turns herself to address me.

La Contessa isn't all she appears to be. Her fingers may be extensively knuckled with an array of decadent rings; her neck hung with impressive ropes of pearls and pendants, blue and white enamelled things reminiscent of medals, or obscure orders; and she might be surrounded in the room by Regency furniture and paintings of haughty relatives posing in country settings, with featureless children and bug-eyed dogs – but there's something about the place, a junk-shop utility, that's difficult to take seriously. I'm tempted to screw a loupe in my eye and hold her hand up for a closer look, but instead I unpack my bag and get ready for the examination.

The referral doesn't say anything about any of this, of course, but

Rae gave us the heads up. Rae is a physio. She came to see La Contessa earlier in the day, and was sufficiently impressed by everything she said about her life as an actress and scriptwriter, and her relation to half the royal family in Italy, to look her up on imdb. When that failed, she turned to Google, and came up with a much richer vein of information, which seemed to show that the only role La Contessa Eleganza di Dramamine had ever played in her life was La Contessa Eleganza di Dramamine. A role she plays to perfection.

'Now look,' she says – but then instantly appears distracted, tipping her head to one side like an inquisitive bird and scrutinising my face. 'Have we met before? On a film set somewhere? What do you do when you're not nursing? What d'you get up to?'

I'm always a little reluctant to tell anyone I'm a writer. Especially of a blog. It would feel like a duck hunter standing up in the reeds with a whistle, gun and hat with a duck on top. But I'm instinctively honest, and besides, I want to feel like I am actually a writer, and declaring it might go someway to making that happen, even if the next step would probably be to go to a support group, Writers' Anonymous, and stand up when it's my turn, and say Hi. I'm Jim, and I'm a writer.

'I write,' I tell her, a little forlornly.

'Fabulous!' says La Contessa. 'Look in the drawer to my right, would you?'

The drawer is filled with business cards. I'm tempted to shuffle through them and see if they all say the same thing, but instead I take the first one I lay my hands on, and hold it up. A fancy gilt affair, curly lettering, La Contessa's name followed by a long line of acronyms.

'Send me some of your work,' she says. 'It's all about the contacts, you know.'

'Great! Thanks!' I say, putting it in my pocket.

'This back pain really is the most dreadful nuisance. I'm halfway through a project and it's cutting across everything like mad.'

'What's the project?'

'Oh – you'd love it! It's called The Heart is Another Country. It's about a Mata Hari figure in World War One who has to choose between duty to her country and this rather scrumptious German general she falls in love with. It's in pre-production, but not quite cast. Darling Judi is frightfully keen to play the mother. Do you know Judi?'

'Dench?'

'That's the one!' says La Contessa. 'Stephen wants to play the general, but I don't know how to put him off. He's frightfully brilliant, of course, and he looks marvellous in moustaches, but I'm just not sure I could take him seriously.'

❧

Joan is sitting in the sunshine on an antique walnut chair, an aluminium walking stick planted squarely in front of her, both hands resting on it, giving her the appearance of a graven warrior leaning on a sword. I have to say she'd look pretty good in a helmet, with a nose-piece and slits for eyes; as it is, her only armour is a tweed skirt, silk blouse and metallic hairdo.

And if Joan is a warrior, her declared enemy would be Sciatica.

'I'm a martyr to it,' she says, thumping her stick on the carpet twice, which she does periodically, to emphasise the key points.

'Not that I let it win. I know what you, the doctor and everybody else will say. You've got to keep moving Joan. Physiotherapy and pain relief, that's the ticket. But all these pills and potions turn me into an absolute zombie, dragging myself around the place, moaning and carrying on. And when I'm in that state I'm afraid all I really need is shooting.

Thump, thump.

'I must tell you something, though. You'll like this. My friend Agnes came round the other day. She visits every now and again. Like the flu. She wanted me to drive her to the mobility shop to help her choose a three-wheeled walker. I said can't you just order it online like everyone else? But she hasn't the faintest idea what online means. She thinks it's something to do with the railway. Still, I don't mind the odd excursion. I drive, of course. Everything's a fuzz close up, but so long as the sun's high enough I get by. So we drove over to the mobility shop, and spent an absolute lifetime looking at their range. I suggested the most solid looking thing with a basket on the front and a seat to sit on if it came to that. But Agnes being Agnes she went for the racy red affair, a three-wheeler, something that wouldn't look out of place at Brands Hatch. Whilst she was fiddling around with a cheque book – a cheque book! I mean, honestly. She's like something out of the Middle Ages! – Anyway, whilst she was driving the assistant absolutely insane with her chaotic bag and her endless requests, I took the opportunity to nip next door to the paper shop to get my copy of the Financial Times. Whilst I was in there chatting to the shopkeeper about call centres or somesuch, a woman came into the shop and asked me if I knew a woman with a red three-wheeled walker. So I said Yes, I'm afraid I do. So she said Well she's just fallen over!'

Thump, thump.

Pine Close is a tributary of a dozen streets, everything leading off from everything else in repeating patterns like a fractal maze, the town planning equivalent of a fern or maybe an ice crystal. All the streets are named after trees, which is odd, because actually there are no trees here at all, excepting one or two brutalised sticks at best, and a scattering of drought-tolerant shrubs. The only characteristic the estate shares with a forest is that it's easy to get lost. All of the houses are identical, a monotonous procession of red-bricked buildings, shoulder-to-shoulder behind iron railings, green and black and blue bins, cars parked in numbered bays, the only thing to differentiate each from each maybe a variation in the way the net curtains are hung, a plastic heron or a planter with a blob of box and a solar-powered night light, and a sign on the corner of each group to tell you how the numbers are running. I half expect to see a giant hand reach in to push a car around the turning circle, stop, open the boot and pinch out shopping bags of tiny, ultra-realistic shopping.

To add to the unreality of it all, I've come to collect a leg.

'Sorry to ask you,' says Lucy, one of the senior OTs. 'Only it got left behind when Bill went into hospital. Now he's gone to rehab and he needs it. There's a keysafe, so all you've got to do is pick it up and take it to Bevan House.'

I'm slow to read the numbers, attracting the suspicious gaze of three elderly people standing on the corner. They can see my uniform, so I'm hoping they'll guess I'm legit – although by the way they stare at me, it's like they think I've bought the kit off eBay and I'm scouting for mischief.

'Morning!' I say through the open window of the car as I crawl past.

They stare at me and say nothing.

I park in a space marked with a V (for Villain, judging by the looks I get from the trio), take my diary, and walk along the path in the direction of Bill's house.

I knock on the door, just in case there's anybody there, and then start fiddling with the keysafe, which doesn't seem to work. Then I notice another keysafe, a newer, nicer one, to the other side of the door. I'm just replacing the cover of the old one when a back gate opens and an elderly man appears. His face has a slack and aggrieved look.

'What are you doing?' he says.

'Oh! Hello!' I say. 'I'm Jim, from the hospital. I've come to collect Bill's leg.'

'Who did you say you were?'

'Jim. From the hospital.'

'Bill's not here.'

'No. I know.'

'He's in the hospital.'

'Yes. Well – no. Actually – he's just been transferred to a nursing home.'

'Who did you say sent you?'

'The hospital.'

The man frowns and pulls back, keeping his hand on the gate.

Meanwhile, the three people who'd been standing at the corner have migrated to the railings behind me.

'What's going on, Ted?' says one of them, a woman in a hat that looks like a tea cosy.

'He says he's come to see Bill.'

'Bill's in hospital,' says the woman.

'He's been there weeks' says one of the others, an elderly man with a walking stick that he taps on the ground a couple of times. 'I saw them take him away. In an ambulance.'

'What do you want?' says tea cosy woman. 'Who sent you?'

I hold up my pass, feebly, an atheist waving a crucifix.

'I'm Jim, from the community health team. Bill's been transferred to a nursing home and they asked me to collect his leg.'

'His leg?'

'Yes. He's an amputee.'

I'm suddenly stricken with the thought I've got the wrong Bill.

'He'll need that,' says the other of the three, a bored looking man in a voluminous duffle coat. I smile at him, playing my advantage.

'So let's get this straight,' says Ted. 'The hospital asked you to come and fetch Bill's leg because he needs it at the hospital. Is that right?'

'The nursing home. Yes. I think they want to start rehabilitation. I'm sorry but – are you a relative?'

'His brother,' says the man, straightening. 'Why?'

'Patient confidentiality. Can't say too much.'

Which sounds ridiculous, even to me. I don't think it's helped.

'Bill doesn't have any secrets from me,' says Ted.

'No, no. That's not what I meant. Anyway – look – sorry – we've got off on the wrong foot,' I tell him, holding out my hand. 'Ironically.'

'Why were you fiddling around with the keysafe if Ted was there?' says tea cosy woman.

'Well I didn't know that, did I?'

'You could have knocked. That's what people generally do, you know?'

'I did knock.'

'Not very loudly,' says Ted. 'It was like you didn't want anyone to hear.'

'Did you hear that?' says tea cosy woman, turning to stick man.

'Hear what?'

'He didn't want anyone to hear.'

'Oh' says stick man, but he looks confused, and he taps his stick again.

'So – do you live here, too?' I say to Ted, as innocently as I can.

'No. I just came round to have a tidy up.'

'That's nice of you. I don't suppose you came across a leg, did you?'

'Of course I did. It's in the conservatory.'

'Would you mind if I took it, then? Only...' I smile and shrug and hold my diary up, in a mime that's supposed to illustrate how busy I am, what a day, etc, etc. But it's a tough crowd and they don't say anything.

Ted purses his lips and shakes his head, as if this is the most unsatisfactory thing that's ever happened to him.

'You don't have to give me the leg if you don't want to,' I tell him, hoping it'll take the pressure off and make him more compliant. 'I'll just tell them at the nursing home and they can make other arrangements.'

'Like what?' chips in duffle coat man. 'He needs his leg.'

'Exactly!'

'Come on, then,' says Ted, sighing and retreating. 'But I'm not happy.'

A couple of minutes later I'm walking back up the path holding Bill's leg. It's a below-the-knee amputation, so the leg consists of a large, silicone cup and stocking, an aluminium strut, and a plimsoll on the foot. I carry it in front of me in a self-conscious way, like an Olympic runner holding the flaming torch, making my way through the crowds.

'Don't drop it,' says duffle coat man. 'It'll run off.'

∽

Isla is sitting with her stork legs up on a stool, watching telly. It's another property programme, the kind where stressy couples are helped to find somewhere to live. I don't know where this particular couple have gone – maybe to weep in the garden – but the experts, a man in a tailored beard and mohair coat, and a woman in primary colours and teeth so white they look like gum shields, are sauntering shoulder-to-shoulder down the hall, the man being enthusiastic about the coving, the woman scathing about the electrics.

'Look at him!' says Isla. 'Who'd buy a house off him?'

'I wouldn't buy a coat.'

'My husband was handy with a screwdriver.'

'Was he?'

'He'd sort that place out in no time.'

'Sounds like someone to know.'

'That's why I married him. One of the reasons. Now then. What have you come to do? More blood, I expect. Why's everyone so interested in my blood? What's so special about it?'

'They just want to see how your kidneys are doing.'

'My kidneys? I'm ninety-five. How d'you think my kidneys are doing?'

'Quite. Still – you can always refuse. You don't have to have these things done, Isla. Just so long as you understand what it is you're refusing.'

'Oh I understand alright. I understand all too well. Come on if you're coming, then. You've got a job to do. I don't want to get you in trouble.'

She bunches up her sleeve and stares at the telly whilst I set up.

'What did you do before you retired?' I ask her.

'I was a writer, dear.'

'Oh really? What did you write?'

'They were called partworks. I don't suppose you know.'

'Isn't it where you buy a magazine every month on a particular subject? And you get stuff with it, like bits of a model car or a boat or something, and you gradually put it all together, until by the end you've got a model of the Ark Royal that cost pretty much the same as the original.'

'You've got it! A friend of mine did one about planes. You'd get a sweet little balsa wood version, which looked quite fun to chuck around outside but mine always crashed first time, so it was a bit of a swizz.'

'Did you have a specialist subject?'

'Not really. Fashion. Arts and Crafts. Hobbies, that sort of thing. Knitting. It paid the bills, and I liked digging around in the library. Ouch! That smarts!'

'Sorry.'

'I thought you were supposed to say sharp scratch? I should know. I've watched enough hospital programmes.'

'I thought I'd get you whilst you were distracted.'

'Well it didn't work, did it?'

'No.'

'Maybe I should write something about nursing and you should read it.'

'Every little helps.'

Isla's friend June coo-ee's, knocks and breezes in. She's as emphatically made-up as the housing expert on TV, with orange lipstick, tan coloured foundation that ends in a line just below the chin, and hair that seems to stay pointing forwards when she turns to close the door behind her.

'Just thought I'd pop by,' she says. 'I didn't know you had company...'

'I don't,' says Isla. 'He's taking blood.'

'Oh. Well. That's nice. I won't get in your way.'

'New blouse?' says Isla, rolling up her sleeve and buttoning the cuff.

'Yes! Do you like it, Isla? I got it at the market. I was worried it might look a bit hippyish. And I wasn't sure about the fit. You can't really try these things on there, can you? Not with everyone walking by.'

She smiles at me, like she's just caught me walking by. I blush.

'Paisley,' says Isla.

'Yes! That's right!' says June. 'Gosh – don't you know a lot about a lot? Isla used to be a writer,' she says to me.

'Yes. She was just saying.'

'Persian,' says Isla. 'The pattern, I mean.'

'I thought it was Scottish.'

'That's just where they started making them in the eighteen hundreds or thereabouts. The soldiers brought back shawls from the East Indies, and the Paisley weavers copied the design.'

'Oh! How fascinating!' says June, smiling at me so broadly her lipstick crackles. 'Isn't that wonderful?'

'Did you keep the receipt?' says Isla.

∽

'What's the verdict, doc? Still alive? You can tick that box, then. But I can tell you what the problem is, without none of your fancy nonsense. I'm ninety-four! Yes! That's what the problem is. Ninety-four and fucked, 'scuse my French. We're all living too long, y'see? Weren't too long ago I'd have popped off by now. But we're all hanging around in limbo and no fucker knows what to do with us and I don't see no end to it – d'you? I don't mind, though. I've had my life. I was in Germany, just after the war. You talk about hard times now, but you should 'a seen it back then, mate. Terrible. All them kids, scratching around the ruins for someink' to eat. We did that, and worse. Bodies everywhere. I'd never seen nuffin' like it. People talk about war like it's something grand, something to be proud of. I weren't proud. Far from it. I still have the dreams. But then again, y'see, I was just a kid myself, twenty years old and no sign of a razor. We lived day to day, though. We went dancing and tried to forget about all the bad stuff. It's just the way it was and that was that. There weren't nothing you could do about it. When I made it back home for good I followed the family trade. In the theatre. I weren't a hoofer like me ol' man.

Nah! I liked all the backstage stuff, the lighting mainly. Dad was the real thing, though, a proper West Ender. He had this nice little thing going with Gertrude Lawrence. You've heard of her, I suppose? They did pretty well, but then she nicked off to America and and he ended up stage doorman at the Winter Gardens. Still, she never forgot him. When she come back he was the first one she'd look up. She'd be outside knocking on the door in her pearls and furs and mum'd be shouting up the stairs Oi Billy, your fancy bird's back! I loved it in the theatre, though. I was at home there. It was in me blood. I remember one day, I was sitting out front watching them sort out the flats, and Alec Guinness was sitting next to me with his feet up. And he says to me Jack. Look at me. I've got no legs to speak of. I'm losing my hair. I've been working myself 'alf to death and still I 'int got ten shillings to me name. What are my chances, d'you think? But I set him straight pretty quick. That was an easy one. I mean – c'mon! Alec Guinness!'

Elsa has a history of falls and unexplained blackouts, so when she doesn't answer the phone I drive straight over to investigate.

The house is a low white building set back from the road, a dark garden to one side with contorted sculptures dotted about and random things strung from branches, giving the place a watchful, witchy feel. I fetch the key from the keysafe and let myself in.

Hello? It's Jim, from the hospital...

There's uncollected post right by the door. I pick it up and put it on a stool.

Hell...oooo.

Nothing.

Last time I was here the house was full. There was Elsa's husband, Freddy, his carer, a carer for Elsa, and then two therapists whose visits had unexpectedly clashed. Freddy had been shuffling excitedly up and down the hallway, stirred by all the commotion, presenting random things after looking for them with great enthusiasm, tugging on his braces, marching on the spot in his slippers like a seagull paddling for worms. Elsa had been the quiet centre of it all, sitting on an armchair in her nightie, overwhelmed.

Now the hallway is silent, what little light there is reflecting dully off the parquet flooring.

Hell...ooo. It's Jim ... from the hospital...

Every door leading off from the hallway is shut, which I take as a sign the place is empty. Still, I have to open each one and check that Elsa isn't on the floor.

Kitchen.

Bathroom.

Closet – (a shock, to be confronted by coats on hooks, close-up).

Which leaves the door to the sitting room at the furthest end of the hallway.

Hell...ooo.

I knock and open the door.

Utterly silent except for the honeyed tocking of a longcase clock. A saturating green light spills in from the garden through the patio windows illuminating an empty leather sofa, dark paintings on the walls, a carved mirror and dining table, a leather bucket armchair with its back to me. And as if my entrance has stirred everything up, the clock suddenly gives a shuddery kind of cough and a kick, and starts grinding out the quarter. And that's when Freddy decides to swing round in the bucket armchair, his hands spread, his eyes wide.

'Oh my Jesus Christ!' I say, falling back.

'Har hah!' says Freddy.

It helps they have a picture of Tarzan on the wall.

'Is that Ron Ely?'

'Where?'

Brenda glances towards the door, but I point to the dresser, the side of it, and a rather tatty colour photo stuck there with tape. Brenda gets up stiffly and shuffles over to look.

'Oh – him? No. That's erm... that's Lex Barker.'

'Oh! I thought it was Ron Ely. The TV Tarzan.'

'No. It looks a bit like Ron Ely. But it's not. It's Lex Barker.'

'I've never heard of Lex Barker.'

'You've never heard of Lex Barker?'

'No.'

Brenda leans forwards and shouts in the direction of her sister.

'Jean? Did you hear that? Jean?'

Jean has fallen asleep in the chair – although she's so slumped forward powered-off might be a better description. Her chin is resting on her cardigan, and she's breathing in slow, regular breaths that puff out her toothless cheeks and escape with a soft, soughing kind of noise through her lips.

'What?' she says, straightening alarmingly, paddling her arms and legs. 'I must've dropped off.'

'Never mind,' says Jean, and painfully turns, and sits back down again.

Even though I've never heard of Lex Barker, he strikes me as a way in. Brenda and Jean have been struggling to get by the last few years, completely off the radar of health and social services. A paramedic has alerted us to their plight, and I've been sent in to see how things are and what could be done to help. So far Brenda has been tight-lipped, offering nothing, answering my questions with a guarded yes or no, the smallest shake of her head. I wonder what's happened in the past to make her so suspicious.

'God! However many Tarzans were there? I mean – you've got Johnny Weissmuller...'

'He wasn't the first,' says Brenda. 'There was one just after the war. Elmo Lincoln.'

'Who?'

Brenda shrugged.

'I never saw it. And another one after that. It's always been popular, Tarzan. For some reason.'

'Johnny Weissmuller,' I say, struggling to think of something to say that'll keep the momentum going. 'Wasn't he an Olympic swimmer or something?'

'He was. He came over in thirty-eight, to open the lido in Saltdean.' She turns a loose wedding band round and round on her finger. 'Although how they persuaded him away from California I'll never know.'

'I remember Ron Ely,' I say, looking at Lex Barker's picture again. 'I remember they had stock footage of crocodiles thrashing around in the water and elephants rampaging, and they tried to crowbar them in every episode.'

'Telly's come a long way,' says Brenda. 'They were poorer times back then. No-one had the money for real crocodiles.'

'Gordon Scott!' says Jean, unexpectedly 'He was my favourite!'

'Gordon Scott? You've changed your tune!' shouts Brenda. 'I thought it was Lex Barker! We'll have to get another picture!'

Jean doesn't reply. Eventually Brenda relaxes back in the chair, picks some lint off her skirt.

'I don't know,' she says after a while. 'Too many Tarzans, that's the problem.'

✦

Aggie looks like the police photo of a ruined children's clown finally busted for drugs. All she needs is a handheld name board and number. To the side. Full profile. Washed out, no make-up, hair still out in banded clumps. Dark brown eyes screwed up against the flash. Heavy lower lip rolling out from ill-fitting, tobacco stained dentures.

'I went up that eye hospital,' she says. 'The doctor there, he turns round to me and he says I need an injection. What for, I says. Well, he says, you got that much pressure building up, if you don't have it done soon your eye'll pop out. Oh, I says. Yes, he says. I'll make you an appointment. Well – if you're that worried you think my eyeball's gonna explode, why don't you give me the injection now? I'm here, aren't I? Oh, he says. Alright. So then he gets out this needle and he jabs me in the eye. Not just once, mind. Four times. Four times! It's no wonder you give people a bit of a run-up, I says. It might be a little sore he says. Sore? He might as well have scooped my eye out and jumped on it. Anyway, I was on my way back into the waiting room when I saw this little old woman sitting on her own, looking pretty cheesed off. So I went over to her and I give her an orange. Honestly – she was so pleased. It was like I'd given her the world. I said to her, I said It's just an orange, love. Don't worry about it. I'm sure someone'll do the same for me when I'm sitting there as old and hopeless as you.'

11: Hostile Territory

Derek is sitting on the sofa, both legs stretched out on a stool, a tartan throw neatly draped over his lap – so precisely aligned it's like a draughtsman has lain a grid over the lower half of him pending further work. Derek is cradling half a mug of tea on his belly, only freeing a hand now and again to point aggressively, either at me, or at Mia, the nurse who's come to do the assessment with me.

'Listen to me... just for one second,' he says, in a hoarse and curiously fractured way, zoning in and out, soft one moment and aggressively emphatic the next, as if he's speaking from a great distance and the signal keeps getting distorted, 'I do not appreciate... I do not appreciate...yeah? All this, what you are doing. It irritates me, high up, in here...' slowly transferring the pointing finger to his right temple and tapping, firmly, twice. I wonder if that's the side he had the stroke, and I make a note to ask his wife Sandra about it. 'I do not appreciate this,' he says. 'I do not want it. Let me tell you something. I have been round the world. A few times. I've walked it. The entire world. And I've seen things. You wouldn't believe what I've seen. I've seen people killed. Yeah? You cannot imagine...'

'You're absolutely right,' says Mia. 'I can't. But – if I could just explain why we've come here today...'

Mia is unflappable. She wears her long years as a community nurse lightly, but with great warmth. It's impressive to see how patiently she's able to maintain her focus in the face of Derek's behaviour, not rising to his challenges, progressing the meeting as best she can, slowly and neutrally, her clinical objective always in mind. I feel like a naturalist taking notes on a species of big cat, stalking its prey on the prairie. It's instructive to watch her work, to see how she continually makes tiny adjustments to her approach, the way she sits, the way she puts her notes to one side, the way she holds him in her attention. If she had a tail it would be switching, infinitesimally, at the tip.

'No! Now – wait!' says Derek. 'Let me tell you something.'

'Please let them help you,' says Sandra.

'It's okay, Sandra,' says Mia, reaching over to touch her on the arm. 'We've got time.'

'And you!' says Derek, stabbing the air in the direction of his wife. 'You I'll deal with later.'

'Oh, Derek,' says Sandra.

'You know what you did. You let them in. You know I didn't want them.'

'But you're ill.'

'You I don't mind,' he says, turning his attention back to Mia. 'I don't ... have trouble with women. And I've known a lot of women in my time. You would not believe. But men? I'm a fighter. I've always been like it. Him,' he says, flashing a sideways glance at me. 'Him I would've had outside in a second. In a second.'

'I'm sorry you feel like that,' says Mia, smiling at me. 'Now – look. it's important that I explain to you why we need to see you today.'

'No. Wait a minute. Listen.'

'Derek! They've got people to see. They've got lives of their own.'

For the first time in the visit Sandra looks utterly forlorn.

'I do not want a thing,' says Derek, adjusting his position on the sofa with an uncoordinated lurch and slopping tea onto his t-shirt.

'Oh now look! I'll go and get a cloth,' says Sandra, taking the mug from him. 'Would either of you like a cup?'

'That'd be great. Thanks.'

Sandra hurries into the kitchen.

'Derek. We think you have an infection and we'd like to do something about it,' says Mia, taking advantage of the distraction to strike the point home. 'If you don't let us help you, it'll just get worse and you'll end up in hospital. Again. We respect your decision to say no, and we certainly wouldn't go against that. But you have to understand what'll happen if you don't accept treatment.'

Derek closes his eyes, compresses his lips into a ghastly smile, and slowly shakes his head from side to side.

'Just you listen a minute to me,' he says. 'You've had your say. Now it's my turn.'

'Okay.'

Weirdly, he almost seems to go to sleep, but when no-one speaks, he suddenly opens his eyes again and points at Mia.

'I've been round the world,' he says. 'I've seen people killed. I've seen people kill themselves, but it's worse when they get killed. Can you – appreciate – what it is I'm trying to say to you? The whole world? Because I do not appreciate .... it gets me irritated .... up here. You do not get what I am telling you. I have been round the world, I've seen it...'

Sandra comes back in with a tray of tea.

'There!' she says, handing me and Mia a cup. 'Although what I think you really need is a medal.'

'I've been round the world. I've seen it,' says Derek.

'I know darling. And got the t-shirt.'

'What?' he says. 'What t-shirt?'

'Never mind, never mind,' says Sandra, 'I'm sorry.' And sinking back down into the chair facing her husband, she straightens her skirt and takes a breath. 'So. How far did we get?' she says. 'Anywhere?'

�

'Shall I take my shoes off?'

'No! Why? Why would you take your shoes off?'

'I don't know. It's what I'd do at home...'

'Are you at home?'

'No.'

'Is it raining outside?'

'No.'

'Then leave your shoes on and stop making such a fuss.'

'Okay.'

Masha turns round in the narrow hallway and shuffles ahead of me down the hallway. I feel uneasy, like I'm being led into a cave by a ferocious old bear I've accidentally woken from hibernation.

'Where shall I sit?' I ask her, stepping into a bright and clinically tidy room.

'Not in my chair!' she says. 'The sofa – perhaps.'

I put my bags down, take my jacket off.

'There!' I say. 'That's better!'

Masha sits on the edge of her armchair. She'd be an extraordinary figure in any circumstance – her hair dyed a rich, autumnal red and swept back off her head into something like a horn; her face slack and mournful – but illuminated as she is by the sunlight sparkling in through the window behind her, she seems hardly real at all, more like a brilliant, cartoon illustration. She reaches for a box of tissues, takes one out and starts folding it on her lap, over and over and over, into a tight little pad. I half expect her to reach for a pair of scissors, make a few adept snips, and unfold it to reveal a chain-word. грустный, perhaps. Несчастье.

'How are you today?' I say, throwing my hands wide, smiling as warmly as I can.

'How do you think I am?' she says. 'Terrible. I am terrible.'

'Oh! I'm very sorry to hear that.'

'You're sorry. Everyone is sorry. But no-one does a thing to help. So I am left here on my own, with nowhere to go, and nothing to do.'

And now I learn what the pad is for. She starts to cry – not an open sobbing so much as a discreet overflow of tears, oozing out through the myriad folds of her face, like her sadness was a water table of misfortune, high after a particularly long and inclement season.

Masha has a chronic condition that surgery hasn't helped. She's been in and out of hospital over the past few years, enduring several interventions that haven't worked. This would be hard enough in itself, but the way Masha describes her experiences, it's hard to resist the feeling that her rather blunt way of talking has only made things worse.

'.... an Asian consultant, he appeared at the bottom of the bed with a nurse, and he talked and talked without looking at me once, and at the end of all this nonsense he said Does that answer your question?

So I said no it does not answer my question. I did not understand a single word you said. And I looked at the nurse, and she just clamped her mouth shut, like this... and shook her head from side to side, like this... and then they both went away again. Later on I could hear them all talking about me in the office, because my bed was at the end of the ward. When the nurse passed my bed again, I called her over. I told her I heard everything she said, and how she was a disgrace to her profession, and if I was in charge, she could be sure I would throw her out, and good riddance. And she cried then, and everyone made a big fuss about it, but I'm not afraid of saying when something is wrong. Like yesterday, when I telephoned the hospital to find out why I had been forgotten, and the woman who answered the phone, she asked me what my problem was, and I told her I would not talk to her about it because what was she? A doctor? No – she was a silly little taker of messages who had no business asking intimate questions about someone's health. And please would she fetch a manager, because I would not be spoken to in such a manner....'

And all the while Masha talks, she punctuates her sentences with a little dab of the tissue to the end of her nose.

She talks at great length. Her tone is curiously unsettling – self-assertive to the point of hostile, but with the occasional upward inflection that's pitiful, almost childlike. She lists all the dreadful things that have happened to her, from rude reception staff and patronising community nurses to incompetent paramedics.

'My sister said to me before I came to this country, she said Masha? You will find yourself in trouble over there. But I have never been afraid to speak the truth. I will not dress a thing up just so that people can feel okay.'

Masha pulls a fresh tissue from the box, and I take advantage of the pause to ask if she has any family nearby. She nods to a framed photo on the sideboard. It's a photo of a young woman, forehead to forehead with a horse. On the left of the picture is the enormous eye of the horse; on the right, the young woman, her eyes closed, her left hand pressed affectionately to the angle of the horse's jaw.

'My niece, perhaps,' says Masha, smoothing out the tissue on her lap and starting to fold it as meticulously as the first. 'But she is busy.'

✄

If Mariella was a Tarot card, she'd be Queen of Radiators. You could happily take a photograph of her now and use it for the illustration – a pale, slack-faced woman sitting in an armchair, staring straight ahead, wearing flannel pyjamas, two fleece jackets, a thick, towelling dressing gown, thermal socks and a pair of sheepskin booties. Her throne is flanked – not by cheetahs – but by two large, oil-filled radiators, both on full. Of course, the flat thermostat is set higher than a smelting works. All the windows are shut. All the curtains are drawn.

The heat is intense, a physical thing. It brings you up short, like you just walked into a room filled with super-heated plasma. Blinking brings you out in a sweat. I cannot believe Mariella hasn't expired from heat stroke long ago, but as things stand, she says she's just about coping with the cold.

'Shut the door,' she says. 'Where were you born? A barn?'

I work through the examination as quickly as possible, leaving just the bloods to take before I can go. Reluctantly she frees her left arm from the dressing gown and I start preparing, forcing myself to be even more meticulous than usual because I can feel myself puddling-out at the shoes. If I miss the vein, they'll have to send firefighters in with respirators. Maybe a drone first, just to scope the situation. They're not stupid.

'Hurry up,' says Mariella. 'I'm catching my death.'

The tube starts to fill with blood. Slowly. I wouldn't be surprised to see steam.

'I like the new flat,' I say.

'It's okay,' says Mariella. 'I've got most of what I need.'

'Must be a nice view,' I say, nodding at the curtains.

'If you like staring at people staring back,' she says. 'Which I don't.'

212

The blood is not coming out as fast as I'd like. I reposition the needle. Makes no difference.

'Bigger than the last place,' I say, feeling the sweat standing out on my forehead. 'Plenty of room to move.'

'What are you? A dancer?'

'I wouldn't mind learning how to dance.'

'What sort of dancing?'

'I don't know. Ballroom?'

I only say that because I imagine an immense ballroom with tall windows. All of them open.

'I used to go dancing,' she says.

'Oh yeah? What sort?'

'Just the normal.'

'Oh.'

I have to say – this new flat is quite a bit cleaner than the last. That had been an old building, years past its best, and the crazy temperatures Mariella pursued didn't help. The place had smelled ripe, cooking in the heat. It was like visiting a patient who'd set up home in a giant cheese. And even though this flat is just as hot – actually more so, as the heating and insulation are higher spec – at least Mariella's things are more spread out, and it feels less suffocating.

'Almost done!' I say.

'How much are you taking?'

'Enough.'

An old phrase comes to me. Something about French eggs. Un oeuf is enough. I'm actually going to faint. To keep myself together, I glance towards the door, imagining the delicious breezes in the hallway, the blue sky beyond the balcony, the crystalline freshness of the world.

'Almost done,' singing it now.

'Yes,' says Mariella. 'You said that already.'

Mrs Kerridge isn't at all how I imagined her from the phone call a couple of days ago. Instead of a velociraptor in wig and slippers, shreds of flesh trembling from her teeth, I shake hands with a trim, short-haired woman in her sixties. Her smile does seem a little flat, though, like those masquerade half-faces on a stick – but to be fair, mine probably looks just as forced. We're both doing our best.

'Good to meet you!' I say, holding out my hand.

'You too!' she says, shaking it.

'Sorry for the confusion.'

'Can't be helped.'

'No.'

We stand in the hallway, smiling, swaying slightly.

'Lovely house!' I say, shoving my hands deep into my pockets.

'Thank you! We do try.'

'Amazing.'

'Yes.'

Greg, the equipment technician saves us, wiping his boots hard on the mat.

'Mind if I check the lie of the land?'

'Not all!' beams Mrs Kerridge. 'It's going to be quite a house full!'

We go through to the living room where Mrs Kerridge's father has been installed on a hospital bed. His mobility has deteriorated to the point where he needs a dynamic, pressure-relieving mattress, but because he's non-weight bearing – and a hoist had been ruled out due to the distress it causes him – the only solution is to assemble the replacement bed and mattress next to him, slide him across, strike the old bed and then move him back into position. I'd tasked two of my colleagues to help with the transfer. They arrived in good time, and we stand around making chit-chat whilst Greg puts the new bed together.

Mr Kerridge snr is oblivious to the whole procedure. Opposite, half-way up the wall, is a large, flat screen TV. It's currently playing a Zoo Vet programme. There's a ventilated lion on the operating table, vets in scrubs standing around with their gloved hands in the air, like no-one wants to be first to start.

'A lion!' says Mrs Kerridge.

'Imagine!'

For some reason, what it makes me think of is the last time I'd spoken to Mrs Kerridge. She'd rung the office to complain, and even though I didn't know anything about the case and had had no contact, I was the only one available to take the call. She'd been furious, incandescent. There were a number of things that had gone wrong since her father had been with our service. Promises made and broken. Conflicting advice. Disruptive appointments. It was a list that spooled out furiously as I held the phone slightly away from my ear. And even though I had the patient record open in front of me, and tried as hard as I could to make sense of what she was saying, there was nothing I could come up with that would placate her. In fact, it was less of a complaint and more of an audio onslaught, a release of verbal steam, and the best I could do was lob-in the occasional I'm sorry to hear that or let me look into that for you. The advice in these situations is never to take it personally. The complainant feels aggrieved, so just hear them out, make notes, and resist the urge to promise to fix things that might only end up making the situation worse. It was difficult to bite my tongue, though. I could see from some of the narrative entries on screen that she'd been hostile in the past, refused help and then complained when it didn't arrive, turned equipment away, and generally made life difficult for the therapists and clinicians.

'I think there's some sort of family rift,' said Anna to me afterwards. 'Best not go there. Once the bed's in, he's open to the district nurses, so...'

Of course, it has to happen that the bed is late.

There's a misunderstanding between the therapist who ordered it and the senior therapist who signed it off (it's an expensive piece of kit). So the delivery date gets bumped, and I'm tasked to call Mrs Kerridge to tell her we can't make the appointment but will be there the following day at the same time. I'm fully expecting her to reach through the phone and throttle me, but thank god it goes to voicemail.

I leave a message. I hear nothing back. Everything is eerily quiet. The kind of quiet that falls on a lush rain forest in the lee of a volcano before it blows.

I'm so dreading the appointment I volunteer to be one of the three – not just because I'd feel mean off-loading it onto someone else, but because I'm morbidly curious to meet the woman who's been so vile on the phone, and to see how well I'll be able to withstand that kind of assault in person? It's like feeling drawn to the edge of a cliff to look down on the raging sea below.

But no. Here we are, perfectly calm, half watching Greg assemble the bed, half-watching a lion having its gallbladder removed.

'Amazing!' I say to Mrs Kerridge.

'I wouldn't want to be the one who wakes it up, though. Would you?'

And she nods at me, and smiles.

Like a country that declares war on its neighbours over a mountain ridge, Mrs Alderman has gone to war over her back.

It's been the cause of a great many problems and pain for her over the years, and lots of clinicians of one sort or another have been involved. But there are some degenerative diseases that can't be cured with medication or fixed with surgery, and the best you can do is try to ease the symptoms and find a way of organising your life in a more accommodating way. Unfortunately, Mrs Alderman's response has been to declare war on everyone who has tried to help. Top of her list are the orthopods, who – according to Mrs Alderman – are a bunch of clowns with chainsaws. The orthopods are followed by everyone else who works in the hospital, Consultant to Cleaner, then the ambulance service, Community health teams, doctors, their reception staff, and really anyone who happens to be driving past, and then her neighbours, of course, and most of all, her family.

Her grandson Joey has been staying with her a few days since this latest discharge from hospital. His main contribution has been to restock the fridge freezer with ready meals. Much further than that he's unwilling to go, and it's hard to blame him, really. The flat is an absolute mess, and even if you brought in a team to straighten the place out, Mrs Alderman would have it back in its current state before they'd posed for photos and shut the door behind them.

This sprawling sense of chaos and complaint seems to attach itself to any contact with Mrs Alderman. I'd been sent in to conduct the initial assessment, which is essentially a fact-finding mission, to see how she is and what she needs from us. We'd had a frank conversation about emergency care support, what she could and couldn't do for herself. She'd agreed that one care call in the morning might be helpful to get her washed and dressed; everything else – taking her medication, putting a ready meal in the microwave – she could do for herself. She could get out the chair by herself and take her four-wheeled walker out of the flat, down the corridor and back, so she was by no means immobile. And it was important to take some regular exercise, however limited.

What happens next is that Mrs Alderman is on the phone that evening complaining that the carers hadn't shown up, that the morning carer had done nothing but stand in front of a photograph of a dog she used to own called Rusty saying how nice ginger dogs were, for fack's sake, and then pulled off her support stockings and took them down to the laundry room.

'They're in the dryer,' she says.

'Who put them in the dryer for you?'

'How the fack would I know?'

'Can't Joey fetch them up?'

'Why should he? He's seventeen! And anyway, even if he did he can't put them on for me, can he? And I can't. Not with my back. I thought you were supposed to be facking helping...'

The carer isn't around to ask about any of this. My suspicion is that Mrs Alderman removed her own stockings and took them to the laundry room herself, but the Coordinator is worried.

'It might be easiest if you just go there tonight and sort her out,' she says. 'And try to clarify the situation whilst you're there.'

There's just one person in the laundry room, an ancient woman bent over a broken plastic trug, busy shovelling the contents into a machine. She looks up when I come in, supporting herself on one arm so precariously she looks in imminent danger of pitching head-first into the washing machine.

'Hello,' I say. 'I'm Jim, from the community health team at the hospital. I've just come to pick up Mrs Alderman's washing and take it up to her. I think she left it in the dryer.'

The woman straightens.

'Oh! She's got you running around now, has she?'

I smile and shrug.

'That's her lot, there,' she says, nodding at another plastic trug, piled up with dressing gowns and throws and things and two blue support stockings artfully draped on top.

'She puts too much in,' says the woman, tightening the scarf round her head, then leaning back into her load.

When I knock and struggle through into Mrs Alderman's flat, the TV is on full volume. She's watching a film – marines fighting alien invaders or something. A helicopter gets blown to bits and there's a close up of Aaron Eckhart looking worried.

'Put it down there,' shouts Mrs Alderman to me, as if we were under fire, too, pointing the remote at an undifferentiated heap of crap in the middle of the room.

'Fack me, I don't know,' she says, muting the TV. 'One minute it's Sense and Sensibility, the next it's facking aliens.'

Donald sits low in the armchair, his left leg bouncing up and down like a jackhammer, his left arm in a sling, his right hand restlessly picking at the chair fabric. However neutrally or sympathetically I try to phrase my questions to gauge what he needs since his discharge home, it's impossible to get a straight or reasonable answer. I'm not making progress.

I have to say I've never met anyone quite so burned-up with fury – or anyone whose eyebrows angled up in the middle so perfectly. It's like his nose is the prow of a bony ship, and the eyebrows are the arms of a cantilever bridge raising to let it through. His eyes are in sync, too; closing as the eyebrows go up, as if he's reading his diatribes on the back of his eyelids, like an autocue.

At least Don's environment is fine. Potted plants. Laminate flooring. An enormous flat screen TV. Donald muted it when we came in, but the show he was watching continues to play. I think it's one of those how things are made programmes, this episode all about buttons. Pastel buttons, tartan buttons, spotty buttons, two-holes, four-holes.... The manufacturing process is complex and fascinating. About a million buttons pouring into some kind of steaming bath, then rolling out on a conveyor belt. What for? Do we need this many buttons in the world...?

'...all you bureaucrats, trying to reduce everything to a simple yes or no, clicking your little keys, ticking your little boxes. Life doesn't work like that. Pain certainly doesn't. Pain doesn't conform to your pissy rules. If I say yes I can do that, you'll put down yes, and you'll say he can totally do that – he's fine, we can leave him alone. But the fact is sometimes I can and sometimes I can't. It costs me enormous levels of pain and suffering just to get out of the chair. You don't know what it's like. I used to be a bodybuilder. I used to be fifteen stone, built like a brick shithouse. I've got a toleration for pain your brain could never conceive of, never conceive. I've got an IQ that's in the top one percent. I know what you're talking about, so don't try to fool me. I know what's behind your words. I can't be bought off like the rest of them. And just because I refuse to be bullied into accepting things that aren't right, I get stigmatised and put down as difficult...'

I'm so glad I'm doing this assessment with Agnes. She's so

experienced and battle-hardened, I couldn't feel better about it if I was an elf on the ramparts of Helm's Deep watching the orcs approach with ladders, and Gandalf was holding my hand.

'I'm sorry to have to ask you these things,' I say to Don. 'I know it's a bit one size fits all. But we need to get a rough idea what we can do to help. Like physiotherapy, for example. Do you think you might benefit from some?'

The eyebrows flick up; the eyes close.

'Oh? Yeah? Physiotherapy? You try living with the pain I've got. You try doing their little exercises. Me just scratching my head is like you running a marathon. Physiotherapy! And what will they do? They'll come and they'll sit where you are and they'll say Oh, Donald, if you don't do anything you'll get this and that. You'll get muscle wastage, deconditioning, ligament contracture.... Bullshit! They don't know what it's like to suffer like this. They wouldn't last five seconds.'

'And where was your fracture again? It's on the system somewhere, but if you could just tell me...'

Eyebrows up.

'What's the point? You wouldn't understand. I've got a better understanding of anatomy and physiology than the surgeons. That's why they didn't like me. They couldn't get rid of me quick enough. I knew their language. I knew what they were up to.'

'Try me. Just – you know – the basics.'

He sighs, then winces, fiercely and dramatically, as if that simple exhalation of breath was the most exquisite form of torture. And then when he's recovered from that, and re-found the energy and the deep spiritual reserves required to continue talking, the eyebrows go up again, and the eyelids come down.

'I have a type two coracoid process fracture distal to the coracoclavicular ligament. Yeah? Know what that is? Thought not. Just put busted shoulder. What's the point of talking about physiotherapy if you don't even know what it is I've got?'

'The thing is, Don – I know this is difficult for you...'

'Oh! You know, do you? How do you know? Been through it

yourself, have you?'

'What I mean is – I can see how distressed you are and from that I can guess how difficult you're finding it...'

'This is the problem,' he says, eyebrows up, lids down. 'This is the problem, right there. Everyone thinks they know but everyone in fact doesn't know. Everyone knows precisely jack shit....'

I'm struggling to make any headway at all with this assessment. And because Don's speech is so overwhelming and so full of invective, and because his eyes are closed and I can get away with it, I can't help glancing at the screen again. Another batch of buttons are going through some kind of electroplating bath, in plain, out golden. They look great. A bit showy, maybe. Still. Nice to have gold buttons....

Agnes takes over. The fact that she's Scottish seems to help. There's a broad warmth to her voice that deflects Don's sniping more successfully, for a while at least. But after ten minutes or so of her best attempts, even she begins to waver. In fact, I'd go as far as to say she starts to sound a little snappy – but then her phone rings.

'Sorry!' she says. 'Do you mind if I take this...?'

And she ups and leaves the room.

I couldn't feel more abandoned than if Gandalf suddenly waved a bony finger in the air, produced a phone from his cloak, and stepped back from the ramparts just as the orcs came over the top.

I turn to face Don again.

His eyebrows are up.

The muddled wave of sycamore trees growing up along the embankment at the back, the viaduct rising high above the houses in a straight line to the heart of town, the shuttered pub on the other side of the road, the makeshift garage with the stack of tyres and the rusting car up on blocks – everything conspires to give this street a neglected, backwater feel.

I'm meeting up with Magda for a joint visit. There's been a

safeguarding raised against Bob's wife Geena. We're here to support each other, to see how he is, how things are today.

'Jimmy boy!' says Magda, tossing her hair back and holding it in place with her blingy sunglasses. 'S'up?'

We talk a little about the situation before we knock.

'I doubt she'll even answer the door,' I tell her. 'Did you read the notes? She's been turning everyone away. Going mad. And even when she lets them in, she abuses them and throws them out pretty quick.'

'Sounds like my kinda girl.'

'The social workers are on the case.'

'Well!'

'She even swore at Pete the physio and threw him out.'

'Peter? Man! That's like being cruel to puppy.'

'I know! So – I'm not sure how far we'll get.'

'You want me to go first, Jimmy? It might be dangerous.'

'Okay.'

'Okay.'

She goes up the steps to the front door and knocks, heavily, like a debt collector or something. We wait a while. She knocks again.

I'm just about to lean over the railings and peer through the front window when the door unexpectedly opens.

A sixty-year-old woman dressed in a hornet stripe jumper, purple slacks and Velcro shoes, frowning at us with a pinched expression. It's like a spiteful child picked a doll up by the face, stood her at the front door of the doll's house, and got ready to shoot her with a BB gun.

'What?' she says.

'Gemma! Hi there! My name is Magda and this is my colleague Jimmy. I'm so sorry to disturb you. We're from the rapid response team and we've been asked to come see your husband, Bob. It's lovely to meet you.'

'I told them. I don't want you people coming round no more.'

'I know, I know. Is problem. But we won't be long, Gemma, I promise you. Just a hi and a bye kind of deal. Trust me. You'll hardly know we were here.'

There's a tense pause that the rumbling of a passing train does nothing to ease. I fully expect Gemma to slam the door, but Magda generously interprets the hesitation as an invitation, and starts moving forward. And really, when Magda starts walking forwards it's very difficult to say no. So instead Gemma flattens herself to the wall, closes her eyes and lets us pass.

'That's very kind of you, Gemma. I appreciate that. Thank you very much, darling. Through here...?'

I follow Magda into the house. It's tall and dark and watchful. A narrow hallway leads off to the kitchen out back, the sitting room to our left.

'Bob!' says Magda. 'There you are! Hello mate!'

Bob is sitting behind the door in a high-backed chair, a zimmer frame to the right. He's dressed in stripes, too, although his are blue like his eyes and easier to look at. Everything about him is the opposite to Gemma. They could be the figures in an emotional weather clock: Bob summer, Gemma winter.

'Hello!' he says, holding his arms left and right like he's known her all his life. 'What's all this about, then?'

Magda explains who we are whilst I get my obs kit out. Bob is wearing shorts, so it's immediately apparent to both of us that he has a wound on his leg.

'What have you been up to, Bobby? How you hurt your leg like this?'

She bends down to look. Gemma, who up to this point has been sitting on the arm of a sofa like a storm on the horizon, suddenly springs up, hurries over, and clutches the zimmer frame with white knuckles.

'You are not to look at that!' she says. 'I'm his wife! I take care of him!'

'Well – yes – I understand this, Gemma, but you know we are here to see Bob. And to be honest with you, unless you have Power of Attorney...'

'I DO have Power of Attorney!'

'Great! That's great! So now, of course, we need to see paperwork. You have paperwork, Gemma?'

Gemma gives a huff, releases the zimmer frame and stomps back to the sofa.

'I'm his wife!' she thunders. 'I say what happens.'

Magda shrugs this off and chats to Bob whilst I clean and dress the wound. I want to take a photograph, but I'm conscious of Gemma staring at me and I think if I do, the flash of it will tip her over the edge. She'll probably snatch up that large, ceramic pelican and smash it over my head, Magda or no Magda. So I finish off with a set of obs – all of which are fine. I can feel the rumbling of her teeth grinding through the floorboards, although it might just be another train.

'So tell me, Bobby? Tell me what happen with leg,' says Magda.

'I fell out of bed,' he says, and then slowly, and irresistibly, he turns to look at his wife.

Glenda's smile is so utilitarian I imagine she keeps it on a hook by the door.

'Thank you so much for coming,' she says – then waits in the hall for me to enter.

'Shall I take my shoes off?'

'Not many of your colleagues do.'

'It's what I do at home,' I say. 'It feels weird otherwise.'

She watches as I slip them off and line them up with the others.

'Easy on, easy off!' I say, although the faux-Cockney falls flat.

Glenda watches me, one hand hooked over the other, a self-conscious and mechanical kind of coupling, like a robot that hasn't had the soft skills upgrade.

'What people don't realise is the toxins they're tracking through the house if they don't take them off,' she says.

'No. Exactly. And anyway – I like the feel of a wooden floor under my socks. So...'

I wait for her to lead me through to her mother, the patient I've come to see, but Glenda stands absolutely still.

'Take tarmac, for instance. They seal it with a cocktail of chemicals that are severely detrimental to one's health. The sun comes out, the sealant becomes tacky, it adheres to the underside of the shoe, and you walk it in. Tests have shown the average household dust carries concentrations of harmful toxins such as PAH, which is implicated in respiratory and other illnesses.'

'I bet.'

'And then there are the bacteria, of course. E coli. C. diff. Klebsiella.'

'Yes.'

'Not to mention all the debris and dirt you'd expect to find in the street and the garden.'

'So – are you a microbiologist or something?'

She flinches.

'No! I'm a lawyer.'

'Oh.'

I shoulder my bag in a resolute way that's supposed to indicate I'm ready to move on.

'You do understand the situation here,' she says, after a significant pause.

'Well – I think I do. The basics.'

'Perhaps I'd better explain,' she says. I adjust the weight of the bag on my shoulder.

'My mother is ninety years old, a fully independent person who lives without assistance in a small village in Somerset called Duckton. She was on a visit to us when she became ill with a urinary tract infection, suffered a minor injury fall, and was taken to hospital, where she spent three days. The hospital deemed her to be medically ready for discharge, on the understanding that she should have one month of community rehabilitation, with therapy and nursing support, and care three times a day. Which is where you come in.'

'Okay.'

'There have been a number of medication changes effected at the hospital, and these have all been ratified by my own GP, who has taken temporary care of my mother whilst she is away from home.'

'Great.'

'Now. What I need from you – other than a medical review this morning – is to provide a report detailing all therapeutic programmes undertaken by your department, nursing interventions and so on, and for these to be communicated to my mother's health authority in Somerset. I want assurances that all possible measures will be taken to maintain her safety when she returns home, provision of all necessary equipments and so on, and continuing care support from agencies in that county. Is that something you can help us with?'

Glenda talks in such a relentlessly steady way that it's something of a lurch when she stops, like coming down a long flight of stairs and unexpectedly putting your foot down flat.

'Well...erm... that's not usually how it works.'

'Explain to me how it usually works.'

I blush, and cast around for a friendly face. All I can find is a vast, frowning, butterscotch cat staring at me from the cushion of a Windsor chair. It looks so severe I wouldn't be surprised to see it reach up and place a square of black cotton between its ears.

'The thing is – Glenda,' I say, swallowing drily. 'We're an acute team. We get referrals from the doctor, the ambulance or the hospital, and we go in, and we make sure everything's okay. Nursing, therapy, care or what have you. And when we're done we refer back to the GP. Or make other referrals for chronic, longer-term needs, to the district nurses and others. And that's about it.'

She sighs once, heavily, as if she'd asked for architectural plans and been given sugar paper with a crayon sketch of a house.

'It's a question of resources,' I say, helplessly. 'A real-world thing. We struggle to look after the people who live here, let alone the other side of the country.'

'As I explained to you,' she says at last. 'I'm a lawyer. Now. A piece of paper with a signature on it constitutes a contract. And your

226

service has contracted to provide us with one month of therapeutic, nursing and auxiliary care needs, prior to repatriation.'

'Has it?'

'Are you telling me this is not actually the case?'

I pick my bag up.

'Glenda,' I say.

She gives a small nod of her head, activating another, thinner smile.

'I've come here this morning to see your mother. To see how she is, do her blood pressure and so on. I have an awful lot of other patients to see today, so I haven't really got time to talk about the finer points of these things, much as I'd like to. So do you mind if we...?'

The smile flicks off again.

'For example. If I was buying a boat,' she says.

'A boat?'

'Yes. A boat. There are certain rules pertaining to the transaction that would need to be adhered to in order for that transaction to be properly concluded, to be watertight.'

An anguished voice calls out from the front room.

'Who's that at the door, Glenda? Is it the nurse?'

'Coming!' I say, shrugging, and holding up my hands. 'Just losing the shoes...'

If I was a comic I'd be dying on my arse. In a tiny, Thirties-themed, immaculately-hoovered comedy club. Three people in the audience, two of them arms folded, stony faced, one of them smiling (the one with dementia).

'I'm not wearing a bra,' says the elderly woman.

'That's alright. Neither am I.'

Tumbleweed.

'Who are you again?' says the son.

I'd been expecting an easier gig. I'd rung the first listed next of kin, a daughter called Louise. She'd been so chatty and friendly on the phone – sorry she wouldn't be able to make it down today, she was caught up at the stables... not in a bad way... horses? who'd have them... that kind of thing... but it was okay... her brother and sister-in-law would be over to meet me... thanks for ringing... thanks for everything, and so on.

Walking into the house is like walking into a wall. Made of ice.

'So – tell me again who you are?' says the son.

'A nursing assistant.'

'Assistant?'

'Yes. Well – my official title is Assistant Practitioner. But everyone just thinks that means I'm a doctor. So I never call myself that – unless I'm ringing a surgery, in which case it helps get past the receptionist.'

Another tumbleweed. Probably the same one.

I can feel myself starting to sweat, even though the room is actually pretty cold.

'Are you registered?' he says.

'No. But I've got a lot of experience, and the rest of the team are just a phone call away.'

'I see.'

(I wish I was a phone call away. At the very least.)

'What team?' he says.

I describe the make-up of the response team. It sounds inauthentic, like I'm reading off an autocue.

I'm not sure which of them is tougher, the son or the daughter-in-law. It's not good cop / bad cop. It's bad cop / terrible cop.

'... so, we get referrals from the GP, the hospital or the ambulance, and we go in and annoy the hell out of people in the cause of making sure the patient is safe to be left at home.'

A tumbleweed the size of a small planet. I wish I could jump inside and roll away, like one of those big, plastic balls. Zorbing, is it?

They're staring at me.

I try to shake myself out of my funk and focus on the patient. I go through the usual routine of taking blood pressure and so on. I use all my best lines. The patient likes it, but Mr and Mrs Medusa just glare at me from the sofa.

'I just need to take your hearing aid out so I can do your temperature,' I tell the patient.

The son stands up.

'Let me do it,' he says. 'They cost two thousand pounds.'

'Thanks,' I say. 'I'm scared of those things.'

His wife snorts.

'Don't let him anywhere near them,' she says, meaning her husband, thank god. 'He left his in when he went for a swim in the sea.'

'Oof!' I say. 'Apart from that – how was the holiday?'

A tumbleweed of barbed wire.

12: The End

It's a long climb up but it's worth it. Peter's flat is meticulously neat and spare, bright as a lamp at the top of a lighthouse, high above the world on this blustery, blue, early spring day. Peter keeps the place immaculately, a pierced mirror over the fireplace, a vibrant figurative painting above the sofa, well-made chairs placed just-so, an oak writing desk under the window, and on the desk, a small ceramic vase with half a dozen stems of daffodil, yellow and gold in the mid-morning sunshine.

'I brought those,' says Stephanie. 'I wanted to make the place look bigger.

'Or further away.'

'But at least we know the desk was always going to be strong enough.'

'Well I think they look absolutely charming, Stephanie. And nobody has to feel the slightest bit guilty about air miles.'

Stephanie is an old friend of Peter's. She's come round to have lunch with him before his big day tomorrow. He's been called back in for surgery. He fell ill out walking in the street, and a scan confirmed what everyone was dreading – the return of the cancer he thought he'd beaten a couple of years before.

'At least they didn't tell me I was riddled,' he says. 'I was fully expecting that conversation – you know – the one where they tell you it's metastasized everywhere, from your liver to your socks, and there's nothing more they can do.'

'Rubbish. There's always something,' says Stephanie. 'You can always go barefoot.'

'You're right,' he says. 'But listen. It won't come to that. Tomorrow I'm under the knife again, so there's hope yet.'

'You see – that's the other thing,' says Stephanie.

'What?'

'I didn't want to get you a fancy bouquet because I knew you weren't going to be around.'

'You could've taken them home with you.'

'Some friend I'd be, buying you flowers and taking them home again.'

'Some friend you are, buying me daffs.'

'It's St David's day!'

'Yes – and St David can shove them up his arse!'

'That's not very patriotic, is it?'

'Who cares? I'm not Welsh.'

'Well you're never going to be at this rate.'

They both laugh.

Marianne is standing waiting for me at the front door, watching me with a pinched intensity.

'Would you like me to take my shoes off?' I say, glancing at the cream carpeted steps rising up behind her.

'Yes,' she says.

I follow her up into the maisonette flat. It's as quiet as a photo in a lifestyle magazine, smelling of floral air freshener and toast.

'Through here,' she says.

'I'm sorry to ask, but I need to be clear. What's your relationship to Jeremy?'

'He's my ex,' she says, 'but we live together. He's dying of cancer. You know that, don't you?'

'Yes,' I say.

It's an unwritten rule that the jobs you think will be the easiest and most straightforward will turn out to be the most difficult.

Looking over my workload for the day, I saw that I was down for a support visit with Jenna, the OT. A palliative patient needed a hospital bed, which meant transferring him out of the existing one, dismantling it, letting the equipment company set up the new one, then putting him back in. The notes said he could just about weight-bear, so there wasn't the usual problem of having to set the new bed up next to the old one and pat-sliding him across. True – the family normally take care of dismantling the old bed, but in this case the partner didn't have anyone to help with that, so we'd take care of business. Another OT had been ahead of us to case the joint, so it should be a breeze.

I didn't read too far into the notes. Just the basics. The patient had prostate cancer. His disease had suddenly progressed, and his care would increasingly be limited to bed. The GP had visited in the first instance and identified what needed to be done. Our job was limited to setting up the new care environment, prior to the palliative team going in.

Straightforward.

Jeremy is lying on his side in bed, one hand crooked behind his head, his legs drawn up. He's so exhausted we withdraw to the hallway again and talk to Marianne instead.

Jeremy's room is small and cluttered, a substantial bedside table with a phone, drinks and things to the side, and a glass display cabinet at the foot end, filled with model planes. As things are at the minute, the hospital bed won't fit, but the first OT hasn't left any instructions about where he wants the bed to go. I can't think he means the front room. The maisonette is a narrow, two bedroom set-up. The lounge is the brightest, most spacious living space in the flat. If the hospital bed goes in there, it'll mean Marianne will be limited to her bedroom and the tiny galley kitchen. If Jeremy stays in his bedroom, though, it'll mean the busy and sometimes distressing business of End of Life care can be contained more effectively. Marianne seems so anxious and friable, I can't imagine her spending the next few months confined in that way.

'I think the bed will actually go pretty well in Jeremy's room,' Jenna tells her. 'Especially if we move the display cabinet next door and put the bedside table over by the window. When the hospital bed's in, you'll have more time to have a think about things. You could ask some friends or family to help with taking some stuff away, maybe putting it in storage. What do you think?'

'I don't understand,' she says. 'What's going to happen with the bed he's on now? I don't want to get rid of it.'

'I suppose we could dismantle it and store it behind the sofa in the sitting room.'

'Why can't we put him in the lounge?'

'I just think with all the comings and goings – carers four times a day, district nurses and so on – it won't work so well. You need space for yourself, Marianne. This room's more than adequate. It's nice and sunny. It's got a view outside. A TV. It's perfect, really. It just takes a little bit of reorganisation.'

'If you think so,' she says.

'I do.'

'Okay.'

She doesn't sound too convinced, though. The problem is, the delivery driver is almost here. If we send them away to give Marianne time to think, there'll be a delay before it can be reordered. Jeremy needs to be on a hospital bed as quickly as possible. The care agency will refuse to authorise care on the bed he's currently on. It's a manual handling nightmare.

'It'll work out,' I tell her. 'You'll see.'

We set to work, moving stuff. It's a delicate job, shifting the model Lancaster and Spitfire planes on their display stands, then crystal glasses, trophies and cups. We bus them next door, followed by as many drawers as we can manage from the bureau to make it light enough to slide over to the window.

'Look at all that dust,' says Marianne. 'I'll get the hoover.'

She comes back with an ancient thing, certainly older than the flat, big enough to ride on, with a huge square light at the front and a cloth bag hanging off the handle. She starts rolling it around, the vibrations of it as brutal as a rotovator.

'I think that'll do,' I say, tapping her on the shoulder and shouting over the noise. 'The van's outside with the new bed, so we'd better get on and transfer Jeremy into the wheelchair. Then we can dismantle his bed and make room for the new one.'

'Just a bit more,' she says.

Jeremy remains as passive as the furniture, but at least he manages to stand sufficiently well to make the transfer into the wheelchair. We take him through to Marianne's bedroom, and gently lay him on the bed. Marianne watches the whole business with horror. I'm guessing that the original OT who'd organised the job had explained what it involved, but Marianne was too stressed to take it all in. There should have been a note in the folder, though. I make a mental note to talk to him back in the office.

The bed is mercifully quick to dismantle. We take it through and stack it behind the big cream sofa in the lounge. It's all pretty neat. We're sweating but it feels like a job well done.

'Like I say – it's only temporary,' I tell her. 'When we've gone you can ask someone to help you find a better place to store it.'

The delivery driver is fast and efficient, installing the hospital bed in twenty minutes or so. We spend the time talking to Marianne, trying to reassure her, finding out what support she has or might be expecting. It's difficult, though. She uses all the phrases that suggest she knows Jeremy is dying, but there's a palpable gap behind them. It's like someone standing on a beach watching an enormous wave curling up into the sky and thundering towards them – and pointing, and saying 'Look! A wave! I must get to safety!' but standing completely still, watching it come down.

'The palliative care team will be in touch,' I tell her. 'They're incredibly supportive. They'll give you numbers you can call to help out.'

Marianne stares at the dismantled bed behind the sofa.

'It can't stay there,' she says.

Once the hospital bed is set-up and the dynamic pressure mattress inflated, Marianne walks in with an electric sheepskin underwarmer, as old as the hoover.

235

'He hates the cold,' she says.

'I'm afraid that can't go on this mattress,' says Jenna. 'Those straps will restrict the flow of air. His pressure areas will start to break down, so it's important nothing gets in the way of preventing that. And I'm afraid it's too much of a fire risk.'

'But he'll get cold.'

'This is really well insulated, Marianne. He'll be fine. And he's got a nice, warm duvet. Honestly, this will be so much more comfortable for him than his old bed. Plus the carers need a hospital bed to care for him. They need to get either side to roll him, and it has to be at the right height otherwise they'll hurt their backs.'

She stands holding the sheepskin blanket.

'He feels the cold,' she says, then walks out.

The next day, Jenna calls me over in the office.

'I've got to go back to Jeremy, that patient we saw together.'

'Why? What happened?'

'Marianne put his old bed back together in the lounge, then somehow dragged him through.'

The old, shadowy, three-storey Victorian townhouse is the last one left in the line to be re-developed. Whereas the neighbours either side are smartly painted and appointed, have patios, architectural plants, chimeneas, vine-hung arbours, off-road parking, the old house staggers on with the archaeological scars of the last 150 years: a dilapidated gate you go round and not through; a rusting iron bench, a chunk of obsidian beside an unmade path, a horseshoe nailed to a yew tree. The whole thing has a blasted, portentous feel, like someone built a family home on the hill at Golgotha – and then realised what they'd done, and slowly walked away.

'Margaret's coming home to die,' says Philip. 'She'll be here in a minute.'

Philip is an old family friend. He's known Margaret all his life – when she was a retired music teacher and he was a child student, come to learn the piano, reluctantly climbing the dusty slope to the front door, little knowing he'd still be doing it fifty years later.

'She's amazing for her age,' he says, putting the finishing touches to the room. 'The only pills she takes are Senna. And you have to crush those up in secret.'

Philip shows me into the room she lives in now – the only occupied room in the entire house. It's been set up as a micro-environment: bed, zimmer frame, commode, armchair for sitting out in, health permitting, to stare out of the window at the busy road below and beyond, the vast bright spread of the city.

It's a poignant experience, standing in this room. The piano she last played a dozen years ago when she was ninety is now an extempore stand for photos and wet wipes and incontinence products. Around it, quietly disappearing into the muted walls, a selection of photographs of ancient vintage, sepia family groups, Edwardians in suits and bowler hats lounging awkwardly on the grass; fading figures in boats or on horses; matriarchs in severe black dresses promenading along a sea wall, fishing boats with sails in the bay; men in huge moustaches and braided uniforms; a woman in a tweed suit and upswept, tortoiseshell glasses, smiling up at the camera, a pen in her hand.

We hear the ambulance crew struggling up the path, so we go out to help them.

They carry her into the house on their portable chair, a decrepit royal on a bier.

'Where d'you want her?' says one of them, sweating.

Later, when Margaret's settled and we've brought in all her things, the same ambulance man kneels down in front of her and holds her hand.

'We're going to go now,' he says, loudly and slowly, 'but we'll leave you in the care of these good people.'

'Let me tell you something,' says Margaret, pulling him towards her. 'You have a very rare gift – the ability to give people complete confidence, and to put them at their ease.'

'Well – that's very kind of you,' he says, blushing. 'Thank you very much. No-one's ever said anything like that to me before.'

'That's a shame!' says Margaret, patting his hand and releasing it. 'Everyone needs a little encouragement, don't you think?' She looks around the room, sees me, and leans back.

'Now. What in the devil's name do we have here?' she says.

No-one knew why Alf was dying, but anyone could see that he was.

And as far as I could tell (it was difficult to ask), nobody knew why he'd refused any of the tests that might reveal the cause, chance of recovery, or time left. He'd been clear about that – certainly clear enough to reassure the medical team that he understood the consequences of his actions, and that his refusal wasn't simply another manifestation of his illness. He may have explained his decision to them in detail. I expect he did. For us, the community health team, we simply had to accept that Alf had declined any further intervention and wanted to be cared for at home. I can only guess why that was. Maybe he knew that anything they tried would be hopeless, and he'd lose his last weeks in a fog of operations, pain, nausea, medication. Maybe he was resolved simply to wade out with his eyes closed, and let the dark waters close over him. When I met him he was as passive as an anatomical doll, frail and uncommunicative, submitting to being rolled and cleaned from time to time, and not much else.

Alf's deterioration had been so precipitous the family had started to gather in earnest, flying in from the extreme ends of the country, and abroad. The home they came back to was as unrecognisable as their father. Everything was in turmoil. There was a hospital bed in the front room, looking like it had been beamed up from a ward somewhere and crash-landed amongst all the fishing trophies and wedding portraits and domestic ephemera of a life. And it wasn't just the bed. There was an abundance of medical supplies and pieces of

238

equipment, the kinds of thing you need to treat an end-of-life patient at home, and beyond that, every available space was now given over to the cause, to temporary put-you-ups, and suitcases, and clothes thrown over balustrades, extemporary family huddles in the kitchen, or the garage, wherever they could gather together, and drink tea, and whisper severely, and let the old family rivalries play themselves out, as they ever will when families get back together for any reason, but most especially now, when one of their number is dying. They'd hurried across hundreds – even thousands of miles – and now they were here they found there was little they could do. Along with their horror of the situation they had to cope with boredom, and frustration, and being separated from their own lives and problems, for an indefinite time. They relieved each other from their vigils at the bed. They did what they could to stay afloat. But the house was an anteroom of death, and the fact that no-one explicitly knew why made it worse for them.

Leah had been the first to come down. Leah had problems of her own, an eating disorder she'd struggled with for years. She tried to encourage her father to drink some of her own supply of fortifying milkshake, holding the straw to his lips, making softly encouraging noises.

'He doesn't want it,' said her sister, Mae, her arms folded.

'It'll do him good. It's designed to.'

'Yes, but he doesn't want it.'

Leah was wearing a strappy summer top that hung down from her, revealing the cruel extent of her illness. In fact, you'd have to say that there was only a degree or two of difference between Leah's physique and her father's, except – Leah was clearly on this side of the line, and he was on the other, and she was reaching over with her little bottle of banana-flavoured, fortifying drink, trying to do for him what she'd been trying to do for herself all this time.

'He doesn't want it,' said Mae.

'But he might,' said Leah. 'Give him a chance.'

Mae was right, though. Alf's eyes were already preternaturally large, made of some dull, inferior kind of glass, whilst Leah's were still bright, and vital, and full of tears.

⟡

It's a complex family situation – as they often are – but the long and the short of it is, Jimmy's been sent home to die.

Although the end has come quickly, it's not entirely unexpected. Jimmy has had an alcohol problem for a good many years, as punishing to his family life as his liver. Nothing helped, not counselling, drug and alcohol rehab, surgical corrections, medication – it all turned out to be a grave but ineffectual chorus singing downstage of the tragedy.

At least Jimmy still has people around him, though. In fact, the house is pretty full. There's his brother, Tom, Tom's wife Stella, Jimmy's stepson Al and Al's little boy, Kevin. Kevin is about three years old I'd guess, a cheeky, tow-haired kid in a dinosaur T and red shorts, loving the drama of all these people, showing off by diving onto the sofa, smashing his toy trucks together, sneaking up behind you, touching you on the shoulder and then running away screaming, bending over for no apparent reason and looking at you from upside down.

'Kevin? Why don't you settle down on the sofa and watch the Formula One?' says Al, although I'd guess that's really what he wants to do.

'No!' says Kevin, diving under the table.

'Don't worry, Al. I don't mind,' I say.

Al shrugs, and carries on unpacking the shopping.

It's the first time I've met the family. Truth is, I'd been blindsided by the whole situation. I thought it'd be an easy call, dropping off equipment and doing some obs on a patient before returning to the hospital to take care of all the referrals that'd piled up that day. When I got there I'd found a patient who was actively dying, and insufficient preparation made for any of it. I couldn't figure out how it could've happened like this. After I'd made Jimmy as comfortable as I could, cutting off his hospital gown to avoid disturbing him too much, giving him a strip wash on the bed and so on, all helped by Tom and Stella, I'd spoken to the office to confirm we were putting in double-up care that evening, then called Jimmy's GP, who was as confused and disturbed as I was. She'd promised to get clarification from the hospital, and said she'd call straight back.

'You've been so helpful,' I say to Stella and Tom as they sit down with me at the table with some tea. 'I'm sorry it's been stressful and messed up.'

'Don't worry,' she says. 'These things happen. At least he's not in pain.'

Tom puts his hand on Stella's shoulder; she gives him a brave smile, then wraps both her hands round the mug of tea, to feel the warmth of it.

'Our son Billy died this year,' she says. 'I suppose I'm getting used to it.'

'I'm so sorry to hear that.'

'I was with him at the end. He was struggling, so I put my arms round him to help him sit up. He was trying to say something, but he couldn't get it out, and I couldn't understand what it was. So I held him like that, and I said I loved him, and then he fell back, and that was that. And that was the start of the year.'

'I'm just going to sit with Dad for a while,' says Al, heading towards the stairs.

'Okay then,' says Tom. 'Good lad.'

'Now you be good,' says Al to Kevin.

'Look at my trucks!' yells Kevin, bouncing up and down on the sofa, smashing the trucks together, head to head. Peeyow! Pow! Kapooooof!

I ring Albert to ask if it's okay to come round and see him. When he picks up, I wait for him to say hello or something; when he doesn't, I say hello instead – but then he talks over me, pretending to be an answer machine:

I'm sorry we're not here to take your call, but quite frankly, we couldn't be arsed. So if you'd like to leave your name and number and what you had for breakfast, then – please – do that, but don't hold your breath for a reply, because quite honestly you're not going to get one. Thank you very much, and goodbye...

I hear his wife June in the background saying Who is it, Albert? – a scuffling sound as the phone gets handed over – then: Hello? Who IS this?

'Hi June. It's Jim, from the hospital. I came round to see Albert the other day.'

'Yes. Hello. Sorry about that. Albert does like to muck about.'

'He probably thought it was a nuisance call. The number comes up as private.'

'We get a lot of that.'

'Me too.'

'So what do you want?'

'Is it alright if I come over and do Albert's blood pressure again? The GP wanted a few days' worth...'

'That's fine. Come over. It's not as if we're going anywhere.'

'Sorry about earlier,' says Albert, answering the door and shaking my hand. 'I get a bit carried away sometimes.'

June is standing behind him, leaning against the doorway to the kitchen, wiping her hands on a tea towel.

'I wish you would get carried away,' she says.

'Hark at that!' says Albert.

'Well I thought it was great!' I tell them both. 'I always swear I'll say something clever or weird next time we get a nuisance call, but of course I never do. I always end up saying Please don't ring here again. Which is so pathetic it practically guarantees they will.'

'I've had a lot of practice,' says Albert. 'I've always been a bit of a clown.'

'Is that what you call it?' says June.

Albert shakes his head, then turns and walks unsteadily to his favourite chair, lowering himself into it with exaggerated care. June follows behind, perching herself on the arm of the settee opposite, whipping the tea towel over her shoulder, then folding her arms. It's difficult to figure June out. She doesn't smile easily, and when she speaks it's clipped and to the point.

Albert and June are a retired couple in their late seventies. June is as fit as you could hope to be – as rootin' tootin' as Doris Day in Calamity Jane – but Albert looks twenty years older. He has a palliative cancer diagnosis, and he's becoming frailer day by day. Symptomatically Albert's steady, functioning at a reasonable level, the pain controlled pretty well, but the prognosis is bleak. It's impossible to say when he'll enter the End of Life phase. One month, six months... I'm not surprised June has her pistols drawn.

I run through the observations. At every point, Albert makes a joke. When I put the tympanic thermometer in his ear (The light'll come straight out the other side); when I count his pulse (So I'm not dead yet?); when I pump up the cuff to do his blood pressure (Jesus Christ! You'll have my arm off at this rate); when I scratch his finger for his blood sugar (That's very nearly an armful).

June sighs heavily each time.

'Just let him do his job,' she says.

'There! All done!' I say, packing my stuff away.

'A-one back to the front!' says Albert.

June folds the tea towel into a square and smooths it flat on her knee.

When I'm ready to go, Albert insists on seeing me to the door. When he gets there, he turns and leans against it.

'Can you give me some advice?' he says.

'Of course. What about?'

'I don't want my family coming round no more.'

'Why?'

His chin starts to tremble. He takes a breath to steady himself, then raps his stick on the carpet a couple of times, summoning the will to speak.

'I don't want them seeing me go like this,' he says. 'I want them to remember me as I was. So what would you suggest I do about that, hmm?'

'It's hard,' I say. 'I know what you mean. But I think anyone who loves you would want to see as much of you as they could. I know I would. I think they'd find it hard staying away.'

'Well. There we are,' he says. 'Thank you.'

I give his shoulder a squeeze.

'Come and sit back down, Albert. I worry about you.'

'I'll be alright. I'll keep on my feet if you don't mind.'

'Okay then. You take care. I'll let the GP know what your facts and figures are.'

'Thirty-eight, twenty-four, thirty-six,' he says, then takes out a hankie and blows his nose.

June comes over and leads him back to his chair.

'Close the door on your way out,' she says.

There's a strange light beyond the office windows, like someone climbed up two storeys and stuck sheets of yellow plastic across the glass.

'Storm coming!' says Helen, standing by her desk, peering out. And she's right – but not any storm I've seen before. Something quieter, more abstract.

'Apocalyptic,' she says.

'I've still got visits.'

She laughs.

'Good luck!'

Down in the car park, I see one of the hospital groundsmen walking towards me. Even though I've worked here a couple of years now, I still don't know his name. He always seems so grumpy, plodding along, carrying or pushing something, an expression as burdensome as his load.

'Looks pretty stormy!' I say, as I unlock my car.

'You're the third person to tell me that,' he says.

His cynicism helps, though. To the groundsman it's all just one more thing to piss him off. I bet if we met at the edge of the world, everything and everyone in flames, a vortex swirling open and sucking the very universe down into its maw, he'd be there, standing on the rim of it all, waving his leaf blower. 'Tossers'.

By the time I reach the patient's address, the sky has taken on even more of a brooding tone. Birds are hurrying back to their roosts, streetlamps are coming on. On the seafront, people are stopping in threes and fours, drawn out of their cars to take pictures with their phones. The lights along the pier twinkle poignantly, bravely, about to be consumed. It feels like we're on a slide towards Totality.

I hurry up the steps to the front door of the house where my patient lives. There's a smart middle-aged couple with shopping bags and suitcases waiting there. The woman is on the phone to someone whilst the guy looks anxiously up and down the street. I'm guessing they're Airbnb people, confronted with the difference between the web description and the thing itself – a discrepancy made worse by the brooding atmosphere of the approaching storm.

'Do you know Dean?' the woman says to me, hanging up. 'We've been trying to reach Dean. We're booked into the penthouse flat.'

'No. I'm a nursing assistant come to see a patient. In the basement.'

'Oh,' she says, and shares a frown with her partner. Patient? Basement? That wasn't in the description. They look alarmed, like they'd been suckered into booking a romantic weekend at the Bates Motel.

Gerry, the partner of my patient, appears after a few buzzes on the intercom. A slouching, elderly man with a prickly chin and squint-eyed leer, Gerry is still in his pyjamas even though it's late afternoon. He stands on the threshold, pyjama bottoms gaping horribly, reflectively scratching the porcine swell of his belly.

'What d'yee want?' he says, distributing a furious eye among the three of us, then glancing up at the sky. 'Jaysus feckin' chris will yee look at tha,' he says. 'It's the end a' tha feckin' worruld.'

I leave the Airbnb couple on the steps, desperately calling Dean again, and I follow the man into the house, on past a yellowing door, down some dark, steep steps into the basement flat.

'Tommy? Here's that nurris Jimmy to see yous.'

He thumbs me in the direction of the front bedroom. I thank him and go in.

There's a feeble throw of thickly-filtered light in the room, illuminating a sink in one corner, a TV on a stand in the other, and taking up most of the space, a dilapidated double bed with a pressure relieving mattress, a scattering of yellowing, coverless pillows, and then Tommy, sprawled in the centre of it all like a cadaverous version of Sleeping Beauty.

'Hello, Jimmy,' says Tommy, weakly. 'How're you?'

Above the bed is an old painting of a racehorse in a shabby gilt frame. It's suffered through exposure to long years of tobacco, but despite the sludgy patina you can still see the flare of the horse's eyes and the sheen on its fetlocks, or whatever they're called.

'You like it?' says Tommy, as I help him to sit up. 'S'moi favourite thing in the whole worl' that paintin'. D'ch'ever ride a horse, now?'

'I did once.'

'Where was tha'?'

'On Dartmoor. It was a sedate old nag called Clapper or something. I was really impressed. We were all in a line, about a dozen of us. And we went down this lane, and then turned into a field, and then the field became a dried-up stream, and that became a kind of sunken path between loads of overgrown trees – and this horse, it didn't care, it just kept going, head down, plodding away. And I thought – this is the most perfect off-road vehicle. There's nothing going to stop it getting where it wants to go. It even refuels on the move. My one did, anyway.'

Tommy nods, then coughs – a horrible racket, like someone turning over an old tractor. He gets distracted looking for some tissues to spit into. I hand him some.

'T'anks,' he gasps.

Tommy has end-stage COPD – a dry description for the curse laying waste to his flesh, to the extent that every element of his skeleton is clearly revealed. Watching him move is like watching a detailed, animatronic model.

There's an End of Life care plan in place, but – incredibly – Tommy's not quite there yet. He's managing well enough, in a shaky, superficial kind of way. Gerry helps him wash, helps him mobilise when he's feeling up to it between the bed and the living room (the irony of that). It surely can't be long before he needs the district nurses and the palliative team with their syringe drivers and anticipatory meds. For now, he rubs along more or less.

'I oughta get some kinda discount,' says Tommy, settling back into the pillows I've propped up against the wall.

'A hospital bed would be better,' I tell him. 'It's much more convenient. It goes up and down and everything.'

'Sure – but why would I want anytin' but my own bed?' he says. 'This is fine for me.'

I want to say that it's better to pre-empt his inevitable decline, because when the carers start coming in for bed care in that final stretch, they'll need to be able to have him at a workable height. It's difficult to say these things without sounding pessimistic, though, so I leave it for another time.

'Okay,' I tell him. 'Let's see what your blood pressure's doing today.' And I replace the cuff on my sphyg with one for a child.

Hans seems too full of life to be dying of cancer. With his bald head, handlebar moustache, fierce expression and thick wrists, all he needs is a leopard skin tunic and he'd be a cinch for a circus strongman.

Hans is confined to bed, his lungs corrupted with secondaries, metastasizing like acquisitive weeds from the seed pod of his liver. When Hans talks he has a curious habit of repeating certain phrases at double the volume, and sitting up a little at the same time. It's a funny thing, like a verbal sneeze. I guess he's done it all his life, because his wife Helga doesn't seem to notice.

'I cannot believe zis thing,' he says, his German accent somehow adding to the strongman effect. 'I cannot! Y'know? Listen. Just the other month I was swimming in the sea in Spain. In *Spain*! Making faces at all the little fishes there. Now look at me. Hopeless. *Hopeless.*'

Helga is putting a brave face on it, though – her and the family dog, Boney, a bichon frise made entirely of clouds, who sits by my bag and frowns any time I take something out.

'What do you make of it, Boney?' she says, brightly.

'Well – vat can the poor dog make of it?' says Hans. 'Apple pie? I say *apple pie*?'

There's a builder's truck blocking the mews. It's up on hydraulic stabilisers as the driver operates the winch, dropping off enormous bags of sand and gravel, the engine labouring as the next load gets taken up, the back of the truck lurching with the sudden change of weight. I can't imagine what building project would require such a massive delivery – maybe one of those basement excavations you read about, an underground pool and cinema and gym, perhaps. A lift shaft to a cocktail bar and viewing platform at the earth's core. Whatever the reason, the contrast with the ancient backstreet couldn't be more extreme. Two hundred years ago these would have been a row of stables with offices, lofts and basic accommodation above; now they're a mixture of chi-chi businesses, full-scale conversions, and the cobbled street curves down right and left not to straw and manure-heaped gutters but expensive planters, artisanal signs and cutely painted old bikes with geraniums in the basket.

We've had to park at the far end by the equipment van that's here to deliver a hospital bed. They could only have beaten us by fifteen minutes and yet they're already half-way through. I'm in awe of their efficiency and sheer work ethic, like scaled-up ants in yellow jackets. A hospital bed is no light thing. It comes in sections, of course, but the main frame is pretty heavy. A feature of the flats in these mews is a steep and narrow staircase running straight up from the front door – no doubt originally to a hay loft. To make things even more awkward, the house we're visiting has a stair lift, so really there's hardly any room at all to get the bed in. When we stroll up, though, they've already got the frame delivered, and all that's left are the mattress, a cantilever table and a few other bits and pieces.

'What did you do – commandeer the truck?' I say to one of them, who is so red-faced I want to lean in and loosen his collar.

He laughs, slicks his antennae back.

'Maybe you could take the table?' he says.

The whole thing is something of a rush job. The GP had visited George late last night. George is a ninety-five-year-old man with a recent palliative diagnosis who has declined rapidly and unexpectedly straight into an End of Life scenario. He was refusing hospital, so the GP had prescribed anticipatory meds, made referrals to the District Nurse and Palliative teams, and to us for urgent review first thing in the morning. Katrina had gone straight there from home and was busy by eight. By nine she'd phoned in to make her report: it was bed care only, so George needed a hospital bed with pressure mattress and slide sheet to be delivered the same day, with someone to be there to help with a pat slide; George needed care support four times a day, double-up; he needed pads, pressure cream, foam lollipops for mouth care – the works. I said I could meet Katrina there at lunchtime to get the whole thing done.

George's wife Valerie greets us at the top of the stairs.

'Forgive my hair,' she says, patting it. 'I must look a fright. But as you can imagine I've had quite a night.'

Both Valerie and the flat have the shocked look of something hit by lightning. Everything is essentially as it was – the pictures, the chairs, the collections of antique pill boxes and books, the Moroccan rugs and tables and lamps, the family pictures on the walls – everything so perfectly placed and orderly the housekeeper must have a tape measure in their pocket. But the furthest end of the flat – the main bedroom end – has a sprawled, disrupted appearance, with a wreckage of discarded packaging, plastic strapping and so on spilling across the hallway, whilst through the open door the sound of construction and the movement of heavy furniture adds to the feeling of emergency. The noise from the builder's truck outside sounds like a fire engine.

'What a business!' says Valerie. 'But you know, everyone's been so kind. We really are most grateful.'

There's a large tabby cat staring at me from the middle of the living room rug. It's as perfectly groomed as Valerie, and I half-expect it to reach up with a paw and pat itself delicately on the head, as she did.

'Grammaticus is very put out,' says Valerie, walking over to him. 'He's nineteen, you know? Like us – old and worn out. He can't tolerate the fuss.'

She bends down stiffly and painfully, scooping him up to cradle him in her arms, just exactly as you would a baby, pressing her nose to the top of his head, rocking him up and down, swinging her hips a little from side to side. He maintains his stare, making little adjustments to accommodate the motion.

'He looks good for his age,' I say.

'Do you think?' she says. Then – still rocking the cat – she looks off towards the window. Down in the street, the noise from the builder's lorry has eased. It sounds as if all the deliveries might have finished, and instead there are shouts and raucous laughter, the plaintive whining of hydraulic legs being lifted, the off-kilter clattering of a concrete mixer.

'Good God,' says Valerie. 'When will it all end?'

The three of us are sitting at the kitchen table. Charles is leaning forwards, propped up on his right hand, his fingers splayed on the magnificent bald dome of his head.

'I know what it looks like,' he says. 'I know I look like a man in despair. But I'm happy. And honestly? I don't care. It's comfortable. That's it.'

His wife Irene sits opposite, methodically working her way through a fat file of notes.

'Charles!' she says, without looking at him, licking a finger, turning a page.

'Like I said. I don't care.'

Behind us, two patio doors open out onto a garden saturated with colour: a fierce yellow cloud of forsythia, vivid red splodges of tulip, diminishing dots of daisies, and in the middle of it all, like the richest and most exuberantly white wedding dress, an old apple tree in full bloom.

'Don't even look at it,' says Charles. 'It's shameful.'

'It's beautiful.'

'Are you a gardener?'

'We've got a garden. I get out sometimes.'

'Hmm,' he says. 'As soon as I've finished this cycle of chemo, I'll be back. You'll see.'

'You rest, hun,' says Irene. 'That's your job. Now look – here's that list you wanted.' She hands me a list of medications. 'Good luck with the spelling,' she says.

There's a radio up on the counter playing classical music. The second movement of Gorecki's Symphony of Sorrowful Songs.

'I don't mind telling you – this is far and away the loveliest consultation I've had in a long while,' I say, listening to the music. 'The last one, I was in this smoky, super-heated flat, all the windows shut, curtains drawn. And the patient was wearing a fluffy red dressing gown, sitting on a sofa surrounded by all these creepy porcelain dolls. And she was puffing away on this fag. And they were all staring at me with the same expression, just waiting for me to faint.'

'You poor thing!' laughs Irene. 'I think you had a touch of fever. But you know what? Some people just like it hot. She must be one of those. A hothouse flower.'

'I like it hot. But not that hot. When I came back outside it actually felt cold. For a while, anyway.'

'Do you remember when we had all that snow?' says Charles, still propped up on his hand.

'When was that, darling?' says Irene.

'Years ago. When we first came here. Or maybe not so long. It was snowing anyway. And I was walking down the street. And I lost my footing or something and I just flipped, straight up into the air, and then straight down again – flat! – on my back. So I was lying there, properly winded, and groaning and so on. And these two old woman came waddling over. They'd been chatting on the street corner, all bundled up, you know? And they came over, and they looked down at me. I can see them now, clear as I can see you. And they said: Careful. Just like that. Careful, they said.'

'Oh darling!' says Irene. 'How funny!'

'Careful! they said. Just like that.'

'And what did you say?'

'I said: Why – thank you. I'll be sure to take your advice.'

I'm in awe of the equipment company. They have an uncanny ability to put a hospital bed into the most inhospitable place. I'm sure one day we'll be called to a lighthouse with a bed seesawing on the roof just above the lamp. Looking around Eileen's small and cluttered bedroom, it seems to me they would only have had two options: lift the roof off and drop it in with a crane, or beam it into position from the transporter deck of the Starship Enterprise.

Nobody needed a hospital bed more than Eileen, though, so it's great they persevered.

Eileen is rapidly approaching the end of her life, her flesh falling away, the most vital thing about her the glassy shine to her preternaturally large eyes.

'I want to sit out,' she says, gripping the sides of the bed. 'I'm sick of this.'

It's no small ambition. Aside from Eileen's general frailty, we'll need to consider the two lines from the morphine drivers feeding in to her right and left, her catheter, the nasal specs for her oxygen. And if that wasn't complicated enough, there's the practical difficulty of the bedroom itself. We had trouble getting in the door, let alone negotiate a complicated transfer. Still, Eileen won't be dissuaded, and (incredibly) her observations are strong enough.

'Hmm,' says Vihaan, looking around.

I'm standing on Eileen's right, squeezed in between a stack of pads, bedclothes, boxes of stuff, a cantilever table, a floor-standing aircon unit, a wicker bath chair piled with towels and things, a life-sized porcelain dog – really, it's more like a storage cupboard than a bedroom for the terminally ill. Vihaan is to her left by the window. A little clearer his side, but not much.

'Actually, Eileen, you know, I think it's not going to be all that easy,' says Vihaan. 'Okay? I think it would be safer for all concerned if you stayed in bed and rested there.'

Eileen stares at him, a little hypnotised. It happens a lot. Vihaan is so striking, with a Bollywood intensity and perfect, crow-black quiff, standing with his hands on his hips, glancing around the place, speaking so rapidly and so musically it's easy to get distracted, like standing by a stream fascinated by the play of light, utterly forgetting you're supposed to be catching fish.

'What?' says Eileen.

'Are you sure you wouldn't want to stay in bed a while longer?' he says. 'Okay? You're absolutely sure about this?'

Eileen turns her head slowly to stare at me, then turns back to Vihaan.

'Of course I'm sure,' she says.

'Okay, then, Eileen. Whatever you say. You're the boss, actually.

We'll give it a go and we'll do our best,' he says. 'But we'll take things slowly, one thing at a time – okay? – and then if anything changes, actually, we'll stop and think it over again. Okay? Okay.'

The hospital bed is in the only possible place it can be, in the centre of the room, the feet towards the door. The best we can do is to cheat it more to the right, making enough space to the left for the wicker chair and a zimmer frame to help with the transfer. It's a spatial puzzle, where you have to move everything in strict order, this then this, or that over there first, to move these, and that there temporarily, whilst you hand over these – careful – back up a bit, then that can go there...

Eileen watches it all pass backwards and forwards over her bed. She's on so much morphine I wouldn't be surprised if she thought the room was reordering itself, flying through the air in a magical, Mary Poppins kind of way. Spit spot. A clap of the hands. Vihaan would make a great Mary Poppins. Not so much the outfit – although he'd be a sensation in that – more his brisk but warm practicality.

'Okay,' he says, when at last the thing is done. He leans on the zimmer, one foot up on the strut. 'So now the room is better arranged for you to sit out from your bed actually,' he says. 'The wicker chair is a good height for you and we've made it comfortable with cushions and what have you. So let us begin to raise you up on the bed, okay? And we'll take it very slowly, Eileen. Step by step. And we'll help you to sit out in the chair for a while.'

She turns her big eyes up to him, and although she doesn't smile or say anything, you can see her gratitude holding there, at some depth, but poised, and delicate, and perfectly true.

Learning how to land

Maybe it was a sign. Maybe bad things are foreshadowed in the everyday, like dreams, and it's up to us to wake up and figure out the message.

It should've been clear enough. When I turned up for my flu jab, the manager giving it was the same person who'd put in a professional misconduct complaint against me a few years before.

It had been a mean, scrappy, stressful affair, but after a tribunal hearing the whole thing was resolved, there was no case to answer, and things settled down again. I started using a meditation app to find a sense of balance. It certainly helped when, a few months later, the same manager was implicated in a bullying and harassment investigation and moved to another trust. A couple of years on I was shocked to hear that he'd been taken back again, but at least it was in another department separate from the one I worked in, so the chances of running into him were small.

Except – here he was giving the flu jabs.

It was just my luck I'd chosen to get the jab when he was on the desk. I was tempted to run away and try again another day, if at all. But then – no. Maybe this was the opportunity I needed to prove to myself and anyone who might be watching through their fingers that yes, I really had come to terms with what happened. So I walked up to the desk as upright and authentically polite as a robot, asked how he was, what horrible weather we were having, and so on, and where has the day gone? and what have you, bunching up my sleeve, making myself ready – for a jab or a fight, I wasn't quite sure.

I blanched a little when he uncapped the needle. He was smiling neutrally and even humming – I think – or maybe it was an incantation? There was that familiar, nub-headed, Lynx-loaded whiff of homicide about him that made my knees bend like a flamingo and my stomach twang. He stood up. I was convinced he was going to jab me in the eye and not the arm.

'Sharp scratch.'

Done.

He slapped a plaster on the wound, a sticker on my lapel.

'Sign here,' he said, sitting back down, pushing the register and a pen over to me.

'Thank you.'

'You're welcome,' he said, yawning. 'I think you'll be glad of it. It's going to be a hard flu this year.'

'Oh?'

And of course, as things turned out, although he was wrong about the flu – as he was about so much else – he was horribly right about the year.

I'm standing in a room marked Condemned. I'm not worried, though. It's only condemned for aesthetic reasons. There are patches of damp in the corners and the paint is peeling off. Whatever the reason, it seems appropriate, given that we're fit testing for the FFP3 respirator face masks we'll have to wear if the pandemic gets much worse and we're called in to staff the COVID wards.

The fit test itself is an extraordinary, cartoonish process, and even though Anna tells me off for making a joke of it '…because your life could depend on this, you know?' – it's hard to take it seriously. I've put on an enormous yellow hood with a clear plastic visor, the whole thing sitting on my shoulders like a comedy deep sea diver's helmet. The visor has a round hole in the front of it about level with my chin. Anna tells me to breathe through my mouth with my tongue slightly forward, like an expectant hound, turning my head to the left, then to the right, then up, and down, and now she's squirting a powdery solution through the hole with the kind of rubber bulb you might use to dust tomatoes.

'Hold your hand up when you can taste anything,' she says. 'It should be bitter.'

I hold my hand up.

'That quickly? Really? Wait… oh… wait a minute…'

She stops, checks the bottles, the instruction on the box, then shakes her head. There are two solutions needed to test for a good seal– the sensitivity solution, to get you familiar with the taste you'll be looking out for, and the testing solution, which is stronger, and gets squirted into the hood when you're wearing the FFP3 mask. You'll only taste the testing solution if your mask doesn't fit. Unfortunately, Anna has used the testing solution first, which is why my sense of taste is a little blasted at the minute.

'I'm afraid that's it for today,' she says. 'Fail! I'm sorry.'

I take the hood off, wipe it down, go back to work.

The next day they cancel all fit testing in our department. The official explanation is that the FFP3 respirator is only for people exposed to 'aerosol-generating procedures', and the cancellation has nothing to do with the chronic shortage of respirators. Instead we're to use standard surgical masks, aprons and gloves as PPE. Laminated signs go up around the place. No-one has confidence in this.

'Isn't a sneeze an aerosol-generating procedure?'

'No. It's only if you're intubating, doing CPR, or drilling teeth. Which we don't get to do all that much.'

'But still…'

Google doesn't bring much clarity. Apparently it all hangs on droplet size – quite literally. The World Health Organisation says that anything bigger than 5 micrometres is a respiratory droplet, and anything smaller a droplet nuclei. The droplets fall more quickly than the nuclei, so you need different levels of protection. None of this is reassuring, though, given how much scientific dispute there seems to be on the subject, and especially watching an enhanced video of a sneeze, how complex and explosively dynamic the spread is. And when you find out that the C19 virus is so small you could line up about six hundred spike to spike across the diameter of the average human hair – well, the fit test doesn't seem quite so ludicrous.

It's academic, though. They don't have enough ventilator masks to go round, so we default to the PPE recommended by WHO. And even that's heavily rationed. The masks and aprons come pre-wrapped in plastic bags, and the little, personal issue bottles of hand sanitizer you have to sign for.

Infection rates among our colleagues start to rise. Bobby, one of the senior physios, a fit man of forty, becomes so unwell he's admitted to hospital. He manages to stay out of ITU, but over the weeks we hear how difficult things are for him, how he loses all his strength, his muscle tone. He used to run marathons; now he can barely make it down the street. Others suffer clotting dramas, breathlessness, chronic fatigue. An ITU nurse Anna trained with dies in a London hospital. She sits at the desk and cries when she hears the news, slumped forwards, inconsolable.

'He was so young. Such a beautiful person,' she says. 'I can't believe it.'

Like all disasters, we made jokes about it at first.

In the early part of the year, one of the administrators sneezed and everyone laughed.

'Watch out!'

'She's got that new virus!'

'Keep it to yourself!'

But as the news got worse and the virus spread, the jokes stopped, replaced instead by a tight-lipped regime of wiping-down – the workstations, keyboards, phones, desktops, even the arms of chairs. The laminated warning signs. To begin with people were awkward about not shaking hands or hugging each other, but the embarrassment faded and there was generally an air of hanging back. More signs went up to enforce social distancing – DO NOT SIT HERE; NO MORE THAN 2 IN THE KITCHEN AT ANY TIME. Alternate desks were taped off with black and yellow tape like they were infected already. Silhouetted feet in the corridors showed us which side we should be. Mask Only areas. A narrowing-in, a closing-down.

Weirdly, our workload got lighter. After a flurry of hospital discharges, they started to dry up. All elective surgery was cancelled.

Families were more available to take care of their own. Patients didn't want us visiting. And what work there was became more dilute, as staff were reassigned from other places. Out of the blue, half a dozen school nurses turned up for work. They sat around quietly, looking lost, checking their phones. There was still talk of us being repurposed, helping on the wards, swabbing in the community, but we didn't hear any more about it and nothing much happened.

The months dragged on, blurring one to another. The figures announced at the daily briefings became as lost in routine as everything else.

'Of course you know it was made in a lab. By the military,' says Deanna, one of the administrators. 'They looked at one under a microscope and found stuff in there that couldn't have come from anywhere else.'

People burn down 5G masts, saying they're linked to the outbreak. An engineer is attacked.

'Well that's obviously wrong,' says Deanna. 'People are so gullible.'

The rota is available online, but there's also a hardcopy available in the office, stuck up with Sellotape on the Plexiglas wall of the Referral Hub, four rows of five columns, each sheet in a plastic wallet, tattered from the constant taking in and out and frantic alterations. Everyone calls it The Wailing Wall, because whenever anyone stops to check what their schedule is for the week ahead, there's an element of prayer about it. I wouldn't be surprised to see a line of candles lit on the shelf nearby, a cardboard dish for donations.

The rota has always been a totemic thing – the relentless, arcane machinery at the centre of the team, pulsing with names and times and availability. If you listen carefully, and put your ear up to the wall, you can hear the wheezy little noise the rota makes: Capacity! Capacity! Capacity…

During the normal run of things, the rota is a piece of administrative machinery that smoothly and implacably regulates our lives. During the pandemic, it becomes something else, something that projects a sense of normality onto the muddle and anxiety of the time. The lights on it flicker as it struggles to keep going with so many absences. But – amazingly – it does keep going.

New letters start to appear on The Wailing Wall beneath the names: SI for self-isolating, sometimes extended to SICK.

The essential work remains the same – supporting hospital discharges, or stopping people going into hospital in the first place. The kind of patient we see does change, though. In place of the cancelled elective surgeries are the End of Life patients, often discharged at pace, with little time to arrange the anticipatory meds, the hospital beds, the double-up care calls. Families and staff are put under intolerable strain. We work more closely with the District Nurses, the Respiratory Team. There's a sense of thinning-out, of overlap, of keeping things together.

As a nursing assistant I'm often asked to help the coordinator run the desk. It's like those film clips you see of traders in the stock market, a phone clamped to their ear, a mobile in the other, waving desperately to someone across the room as they scroll down a screen for some vital piece of data, trying to conjure a workable solution from raw confusion. A cold cup of coffee. A pad covered with mad scrawls: numbers, names. Doodled faces – spiral eyes, crazy hair.

I light a candle at The Wailing Wall and – miraculously – get time off to go to a funeral.

Auntie Ollie died. We knew it was coming but it was a blow nonetheless. COVID is listed as the cause, although she was so frail it wouldn't have taken much to tip her over the edge.

There are only six people allowed to attend the funeral. I don't live that far from the crematorium, so I go along as the representative of Dad's side of the family.

Auntie Ollie was an important part of my childhood. We were a large family exiled to the flatlands of the Fens. The only transport we had were our bikes, although for the summer holidays Dad would pay one of the delivery drivers at the printing works to throw us all in the back with the binders and the proofs and drop us off in the dunes on the North Norfolk coast. Consequently, even though Dad was from a big family himself, we hardly ever saw any of our Aunts or Uncles – which wasn't as bad as it sounds. I remember going to a family event with his brothers and sisters all sitting around the room in a line. It was unsettling to see how alike they all were, clones from a factory that specialised in dodgy, short-legged relatives, the only difference being the shade of dark in their eyes, or whether they had curly hair or not.

His sister Ollie was the exception, though. Her eyes were warmer and more inviting, and though she could be sharp sometimes (there's only so far you can go in denying your genes), it was rounded with a genuine love for us and for her youngest brother. Ollie's husband John was funny, too – a lively guy with a big laugh whose restless leg syndrome gave him the air of a ramshackle cartoon helicopter. Both John and Ollie were stylish, loud, bigger than the life they led, somehow. They had stories – big stories – about running a pub in King's Cross where a police horse stopped by to drink beer through the window; about John going to war, being reported as killed in action, Ollie 'taking up' with a GI, John appearing the day after VE day like a disreputable ghost, missing a shoe, so the GI climbed on the parapet of Westminster bridge and threatened to throw himself off. How Ollie let him. That kind of thing. At John's funeral, the vicar said John had escaped from the Italian Prisoner of War camp and fought with the partisans, and I was pretty impressed with that. Except years later, Ollie told me the truth – about the peach farm and the farmer's daughter. She couldn't explain the shoe.

The other thing that set Ollie and John apart from all our other relatives is that they visited us. Which was a major event. Not only did they have a fancy car with white-walled tires, and bring lots of sweets with them in a carrier bag from the corner shop they ended up running – John drank most of the profits from the pub – but they had an English Collie called Rusty, whose fur was thicker than Ollie's, so thick you could dive head first into it and have to be pulled out by your shoes.

It was always a huge occasion when they came down to see us. A shot of glamour and vitality into the house. I was a little afraid of them but thrilled at the same time. I couldn't believe such people were related to me.

I hadn't seen much of Ollie since she moved down to Exmouth a few years ago. The few times I'd made it down there she'd been weaker, then bedbound, carers four times a day, the garden slabbed over, the car port empty.

'She didn't suffer,' said Barry. 'They didn't allow us in the room because of the virus, but at least there was a nurse to hold her hand.'

I haven't been to this Crematorium before. It looks like a converted Secondary school, the conversion being a throw of clematis over the main entrance, a garden of remembrance and a giant chimney. I'm early, so I sit on a bench in the shade of a tree to settle my thoughts. After a minute though I get worried there might not be anyone else here yet because I'm at the wrong crematorium. So I walk over to the front of the building. To one side of it there's a glass case with a notice pinned on a board: Ollie's name is there, at the top of a list of four, the starter on a fancy menu. I check my watch, look around. The whole place is deserted, except for an elderly gardener crossing the lawn with a wheelbarrow loaded with spades and bags and stuff (although not a body, thankfully). He's wearing a Lawrence of Arabia style head cap, which turns out to be a normal cap with a tea towel stuffed under it.

'Lovely weather!' I say.

'Not if you're working.'

'Is this where I wait for the funerals?'

'What d'you mean, the funerals?'

He squints at me suspiciously, like I'm some kind of funeral chaser.

'My aunt's funeral. It's due at one.'

'What's the time now?'

'Half past.'

'Well you haven't got long, then, have you?'

'But should I wait here, or…'

'Round the back,' he says, thumbing in that direction. 'That's where they go.'

'Okay! Thanks!'

He repositions his headgear, picks up the wheelbarrow and carries on.

Two undertakers appear out of the main entrance, both young, both sweating heavily in black, three-piece suits. I wonder what they think of me, in my cool linen trousers and short sleeved shirt. I feel guilty, and I want to tell them the truth about it – that I've got one good suit, but I put on a little lockdown weight and couldn't do it up, so I had to settle for smart-casual. I know Ollie would've preferred me in a suit. She was always a snappy dresser.

'Can I help you, sir?' says the young woman.

'I've come for Ollie's funeral,' I say. 'I'm a nephew.'

'I see,' she says, nodding, squeezing her eyes shut sympathetically. 'Know where to go?'

'Round the back, is it...?' I say, turning in that direction.

'That's right,' she says, nodding, squeezing her eyes shut again in exactly the same way. I guess she does that after most things; it's probably why they hired her.

They retreat back into the main entrance (what goes on there?); I go round the back.

The path winds round the side of the building and leads up to a big stone car port for the hearse. It's an unexpectedly nice aspect, raised up from the rest of the grounds, overlooking a small, wooded area. I'm surprised. I was expecting something a bit more – I don't know – 'round the back'. This definitely feels more appropriate, something like a ceremonial jumping-off point.

I hang around. Still no sign of Barry and the others. Maybe they're in a car accompanying the hearse. I've no idea where they're driving from. Maybe they're caught in traffic – although lately the traffic's been light due to the pandemic.

An elderly guy in a comfortable, light green suit steps out from the entrance behind me. He has an easy, open expression, made even more friendly by a fuddle of unruly grey curls that flow backwards from his forehead like a cliché professor.

'What a glorious day!' he says, jiggling keys with his hands thrust deep in his pockets, his shoulders thrown back. 'A fine day for a farewell! Hello, there! I'm the vicar!'

'Jim. Nephew.' (Like that's my profession).

'Ah!' he says. 'Welcome! Elbow bump!' We do the awkward little dance that passes for a handshake these days, and laugh about it, which is also part of the dance.

'I expect they'll be here soon,' he says, putting his hand back in his pocket and rocking backwards and forwards on his heels.

'It's a terrible business!' he says after a pause, giving me a sideways look and nodding at the same time, anticipating what I'm going to say before I say it. I'm not sure what he means – the pandemic or Ollie's death – so to be safe I wrap the two up together.

'She died in hospital,' I say. 'The COVID restrictions meant none of the family could be with her at the end. But at least there was a nurse to hold her hand.'

'Ah!' he says. 'Good, good.'

'I wanted to wear a suit but I've only got one and I couldn't fit into it, so I had to come smart casual.'

He laughs. 'Well I think you look absolutely marvellous. And I'm sure Auntie Ollie would've loved to see you here however you were dressed.'

For some reason I find myself talking to him about Ollie's dog, Rusty.

'Dogs are marvellous creatures,' he says. 'I've got a Springer called Dave. Absolutely crazy, daft as they come. But it's difficult to feel too fed up about the state of the world when Dave is running around with his squeaky duck.'

'You're right. I always like it when the patient has a dog in the house. It sets things up nicely.'

'Why? What do you do?'

'I'm a nursing assistant. I work for a community health team.'

264

'Do you?' he says. 'Marvellous! Well done!'

He checks his watch.

'Won't be long now,' he says.

We stand looking out over the trees. We're pretty high up here, the ground falling steeply away beyond the driveway. I feel as if I could jump up onto the parapet, spread my arms and fly away.

'Ah! Here they come!'

A long, black hearse, driving slowly towards us, the young undertaker walking in front, her hat tucked under her arm, the other walking behind with a few more from somewhere, and then Barry, his wife and daughter, and a couple of people I don't recognise. The vicar and I move to the side to make room. I'm not entirely sure I should be standing next to him like this, but he doesn't say anything, and anyway, there are so few people here it doesn't seem to matter.

For something to say I ask the vicar if I'm allowed to take pictures inside the chapel.

'Of course!' he whispers. 'As long as you don't get too David Bailey about it.'

We've all taken our places in the chapel – the relatives socially distanced on the chairs, the Vicar at a lectern-pulpit hybrid. Ollie's coffin has been put on a dais, stage centre with rollers underneath, lit by downlighters like the transportation deck on the Enterprise, with some light blue curtains hanging around the whole thing from an overhead track. I can't help wondering where the buttons to control them are, and what the cue will be to start them. We've walked into the chapel to Judy Garland singing 'Somewhere over the Rainbow', which is a sweet touch. When it finishes, the Vicar tells us why it was chosen. Apparently, Ollie met John in nineteen forty-one just before he was sent abroad to fight. They'd taken the bus to Leicester Square to see 'The Wizard of Oz'. The number thirty-eight. (Numbers seem to be important about this story).

'It was a whirlwind romance,' the Vicar says, 'as things tended to be in those days. In fact, Barry tells me that they were married just a few weeks after that first date. Incidentally, it may interest you to know that the church they married in took a direct hit a few days later and the vicar who married them was blown to pieces.'

He shuffles his notes, as if he thinks there was a punchline in there somewhere but he can't find it, then gives up and moves on to cover his awkwardness with Vera Lynn: 'A Nightingale Sang in Berkeley Square.'

It strikes me that – so far, at least – all the songs she's chosen are from the nineteen forties. I wonder whether Ollie's planting a marker in time, the moment she felt most herself, most alive. Although maybe she didn't choose the music. The last few months she was very unwell. Funeral music would be a difficult conversation to have.

I look around. No-one's crying. Barry is turning his programme round and round, like he's winding a reel of twine. The vicar is standing in a neutral position listening to the music, discreetly keeping an eye on the time. He sees me and smiles, gives me an encouraging blink-nod, then grips the lectern like a practiced driver leaning into an upcoming bend. I check the settings on my camera again, but it's pointless. I know I've taken as much as I'm going to take. Turns out I'm not much of a photographer.

How strange it was
How sweet and strange
There was never a dream to compare...

The music drifts out.

The sound of an electric motor starting up. The curtains judder, glide left and right, click shut in the centre. The Vicar reads that verse about ashes to ashes, dust to dust. I feel disappointed I didn't get to see him click the button.

The whole thing makes me think of The Wizard of Oz. How at the end that embattled, disparate, funny little group – Dorothy, Tin Man, Lion and Toto – how against all the odds and all the witches and stuff, they make it to the Emerald City, to see The Great Oz, when he'll make everything right and sort everything out. How he terrifies them with dreadful explosions and stuff. How Toto tugs aside the curtain, and they see the man himself, the conman, the showman, the trickster, desperately working the levers. How he toe-punts the dog away, struggling to close the curtains, saying Pay no attention to that man behind the curtain! But of course they do, and they're furious, because he gave them hope when maybe there wasn't any. Only – as it turns out – there is hope, and he does have the power to rescue them, because he has a hot air balloon! That's how he got there! And he'll give Dorothy a lift back to Kansas. All the people of Emerald City gather in the town square to see them off. Dorothy's sad to say goodbye to her new friends, but she's glad she's going home. Everything will be fine again after such an adventure. But then someone screws up, Dorothy's distracted – is it the dog again? – and the balloon goes up without her. Disaster! Only – it's okay. Don't worry. Turns out, Dorothy has always had the power to get home by herself. She's still wearing the emerald slippers. So tightly hugging Toto, she closes her eyes, clicks her heels together three times, and repeats the magic words: There's no place like home. There's no place like home. There's no place like home.

She lands back in Kansas.

In black and white.

And everyone's wearing a mask.